LOVESEX

Other titles in the UKCP Series:

LOVESEX

An Integrative Model for Sexual Education

Cabby Laffy

Illustrations by Tessa Gaynn

On behalf of the United Kingdom Council
for Psychotherapy

KARNAC

First published in 2013 by
Karnac Books Ltd
118 Finchley Road, London NW3 5HT

British Library Cataloguing in Publication Data

A C.I.P. for this book is available from the British Library

ISBN 978 1 78049 155 4

Edited, designed and produced by The Studio Publishing Services Ltd
www.publishingservicesuk.co.uk
e-mail: studio@publishingservicesuk.co.uk

Printed in Great Britain

www.karnacbooks.com

CONTENTS

PART I: MIND: THOUGHTS AND CHOICES

PART IV: EMOTION: FEELINGS AND INTUITION

LIST OF FIGURES AND ILLUSTRATIONS

Figures

Illustrations

LIST OF EXERCISES

ACKNOWLEDGEMENTS

I would like to thank the following people who have enabled me to write this book:

- Judi Keshet-Orr, Bernd Leygraf, and Sarah Littlejohn, my early therapists and teachers;
- Boo Armstrong and Clare Summerskill, for encouraging and inspiring me to write;
- Tessa Gaynn and Debbie Pope, for creating beautiful illustrations and artwork;
- Rose McAfee, for the great website design and support;
- my Diploma students, for helping me to clarify my concepts and ideas;
- Scilla Elworthy and Sara Tibbs for reading early drafts;
- Gerry Laffy, Melody Laffy, and Lizzie Ruffell for editorial work;
- Kris Burman, Brendan Canty, Marie Florence, Carole Ingram, Reina James Reinstein, Elizabeth Laffy, Maria North, Alix Sinclare, and Jonny Slater for supporting my health and well-being.

I would particularly like to thank:

- Anita Sullivan, my wonderful mentor, teacher, and clinical supervisor for many years;
- Aleine Ridge, for helping me develop my courses with personal, professional, and practical support;
- Polly McLean, for helping in many ways, including proofreading and bringing my teaching and this book to fruition;
- Simon Laffy, my brother and best friend;
- Shana Laffy, my wonderful daughter;
- Mark Johnson, my beloved.

Thank you all, for all you have done to love and support me through this journey.

ABOUT THE AUTHOR

Cabby Laffy has worked as psychotherapist, psychosexual therapist, and supervisor since 1991. She works with individuals and couples and has facilitated many trainings and workshops. She is the Director of the Centre for Psychosexual Health and has developed and teaches a Diploma in Integrative Psychosexual Therapy. Cabby has also worked for many years as a clinical supervisor for complementary health practitioners working in the community. She is a UKCP registered psychotherapist, a UKAHPP accredited psychosexual therapist, an NCP accredited psychotherapist, and a member of PCSR and COSRT.

I would like to dedicate this book to all the amazing women and men I have worked with, and laughed and cried with, about sexual matters over the years, and to Shere Hite for her prolific work in researching and writing about sexuality and society.

In loving memory of Boo Armstrong, who encouraged and inspired me, and many others, to be the change.

Introduction

Human sexuality is a vast and intriguing subject, affecting and being affected by so many things. It is unique, specific to each and every individual, and it is also universal. Most humans have sexual desires and urges that move us both physically and emotionally. At its best, sexual energy is a free, potent life force that can be used to enhance and heal, bring great joy, pleasure, self-esteem, physical and emotional well-being. It is a creative force, our fire energy and a source of power.

However, in our culture, we think and talk about sex as something we do, rather than sexuality being something that we have and being sexual as something that we are. We talk little about feeling sexual, or the emotional and relational reasons for sexual desire—about the fact that it is usually an "other" that we want to be sexual with. Our focus seems to be on how much sex we can have rather than how we want to express ourselves sexually.

This book is a culmination of many years of personal and professional experience. It is a sexual education manual offering an opportunity to explore a range of areas and issues that are crucial to creating a positive sexual self-esteem. It presents a new paradigm for professional thinking in psychosexual therapy by focusing on sexual *health* and on us all being sexual people, rather than on dysfunctions that are defined around performing sexual acts. It explores many relevant issues and discusses what sexual self-esteem could look like, if we were to celebrate and explicitly value our sexuality. *LoveSex* offers an integrative model for sexual education where you, the reader, can learn more about the richness of sexuality and be encouraged to experience "being sexual" rather than "doing sex" or "looking sexy".

Since my initial training in 1984 as a natural family planning teacher (now called fertility awareness), I have worked with numerous individuals, couples, and groups on a vast range of issues concerning sexuality and relationships. Teaching women and couples about the fertility cycle was originally for those seeking a natural method of contraception, but has become, in the past ten years, more about addressing infertility issues. During this work, I became aware of two striking factors: first, that concerns around fertility were closely linked to issues about sexuality and sexual relationships. Second, that many women presenting with gynaecological difficulties also had a history of sexual violence, which was affecting their sexuality and their sexual relationships. This prompted me to train as a counsellor to gain the skills to be able to work with these topics, and I qualified in 1991.

In 1994, I went on to study psychosexual therapy. This training explored the medical model of "sexual dysfunctions" within a range of psychotherapeutic approaches, and through this I learnt about sexual difficulties caused by medical/health problems and the side effects of medication. Their labels mainly describe sexual desire and arousal issues that focus on the sexual act of intercourse, such as rapid ejaculation and difficulties with vaginal penetration. Inspired by the work of Shere Hite (1976), who has for many years informed us about our true sexual potential and challenged the limitations of our reproductive model of sex, I began to expand this medical model to work with clients on the therapeutic meaning of such difficulties for them. In addition, my own use of complementary and alternative medicine (CAM) to support health issues from a serious childhood illness, coupled with my long-term work as a clinical supervisor for practitioners offering a range of CAM therapies, has given me important insight into the politics of health and the theories and practice of many healing therapies. Here, the paradigm for health and well-being is integrative: treating the whole person, not just the symptom, and seeing all body systems and functions as interrelated.

During twenty-eight years of practice, I have encountered many people who have experiences of lack of sexual desire or arousal, ejaculation or orgasm concerns. I have also met many more wishing to explore a wide range of other psychosexual issues. This includes individuals and couples with fertility problems, unwanted pregnancies, abortions, or living with sexually transmitted infections, all of which affect their experiences of their sexuality and their sexual relationships. Some people have questions about their sexual orientation or sexual identity, or seek support to deal with social and cultural homophobia. Many wish to explore their sexual desires, tastes, and preferences. Some want to discuss their thoughts, beliefs, and values to explore conflicts with their social, religious, or cultural backgrounds. Many people have difficulties with body image and sexual self-esteem, or are affected in other ways by our culture of sexual shame, such as sexual self-harm, sexual addiction, or compulsivity. Seeking help with sexual relationships is a prevalent concern. Many people have had difficult or traumatic childhoods, with a legacy that often causes complicated adult relationships. We have high divorce and separation rates, and many people are seeking sexual encounters or relationships. Others are looking for communication and intimacy skills to maintain and sustain marriages, civil partnerships, or long-term relationships.

By far the most common difficulty I have encountered is the impact of sexual violence. There are just far too many people who have experienced sexual abuse as children or sexual violence as adults. Childhood sexual abuse confuses our brains and bodies as well as our minds and emotions. Sexual violation as an adult can be devastating, too, particularly because of societal attitudes towards victims of sexual violence. Some commonalties include physical and emotional trauma, not trusting self or other, self-harm or addictions, intimacy and relationship difficulties. Many physical sexual difficulties are associated with a history of sexual violence or exacerbated by social or cultural issues.

In 2001, I wrote an article on the above issues called "Developing a humanistic model of psychosexual therapy", published in *Self and Society*. By 2005, this had developed into the first draft of this book, beginning to integrate my theoretical knowledge and clinical experience and developing the integrative homeodynamic model that I present here. I realised I wanted to teach my ideas, and created a two-year Diploma in Integrative Psychosexual Therapy training for professionals, which has been running since 2006. In the past decade, I have worked on developing a model for sexual health, rather than a focus on dysfunction. This model integrates current thinking across multi-disciplinary fields, including psychotherapy, systemic therapy, neuroscience, cognitive–behavioural therapy, complementary therapies, and traditional eastern and western sexual and relationship therapy.

The homeodynamic model for sexuality is sex positive; it promotes the pleasure principle, and challenges sexual shame. Rather than feeling uncomfortable or embarrassed about discussing sexual matters, *LoveSex* recommends that we explore some more ease in our current relationship to human sexuality. Many important attributes of this model also begin with E:

• educational—providing knowledge to stimulate your curiosity and desire. You can learn more about your fascinating and amazing bodies, your intelligence and creativity. Through this, you can explore your sexual potential and reflect, discuss, ponder, and evaluate;

• experiential—encouraging you to get intimate with yourselves, your bodies, your uniqueness and delights. Feel into your nerves and muscles, your fingertips and lips; find out what really turns you on and what turns you off; revel in your sensuality;

• ecstatic—exercises to discover your core erotic themes, experience the free serotonin highs of pleasure and bliss through touch and intimate sexual play;

• empowering—challenging you to choose what you really want and value as ways of being sexual. Choose your own sexual diet, to suit your preferences, tastes, and desires. Experience the difference between "power over" and "power with" models of thinking and behaving;

• existential—redress our cultural shaming of sexuality so we can feel great pleasure and well-being through our sexuality and have a good sense of sexual self-esteem, where we value, honour, and celebrate this gift we have. Reclaim our sense of sexuality from the consumerist dictates of the media, and the advertising and sex industries.

LoveSex has been written for a range of people, such as any one of the clients or students I have worked with over the years. You might be someone with a general curiosity about sexuality who wishes to explore and re-evaluate your sexual beliefs and behaviour to build a more conscious sexual self-esteem. You might be an individual or couple with a specific sexual issue or difficulty that you would like to find out more about and get some ideas to try to change. You might be one of many who have experienced childhood sexual abuse or sexual violence as an adult, who wishes to explore some of the effects this has had on you and gain some ideas and insights for healing. It is also a useful resource for therapists and any practitioners working with clients' sexual issues.

Nearly all of us will have experienced a general level of sexual shaming and a clear lack of celebration about sexuality, as most societies, cultures, and religions denigrate or exploit sexuality. Very few people report growing up with a confident and celebratory attitude towards sexuality and this influences many of our difficulties surrounding sex and sexual relationships. I am fascinated by our cultural sexual shame, why this is, and how it hinders our ability to develop a sense of sexual self-esteem. Shame is like a bully–victim dynamic or the so-called "power over" model, which will be discussed later. The homeodynamic model of sexuality presented in *LoveSex* is more in line with an alternative model of power: "power with", which is central to conflict resolution and new social concern organisations all over the world.

When we feel ashamed of our sexuality we might react in many ways. We might have an increased need to stay in control sexually, or to avoid feeling vulnerable. We might avoid sexual encounters altogether, or sexual intimacy within an ongoing relationship. We might pretend to others that we are much happier with our sexual lives than we really are. We might experience internalised shaming voices from our culture or family and become critical or judgemental towards ourselves.

On the other hand, we might reject this shame and take the other polarity, that of shamelessness, a sort of empty pretence of liberation and ease. In shamelessness, we do not really contemplate the possibility of saying no. Instead, we want to try everything, have a willingness to do anything, the more outrageous the better, regardless of how it actually makes us feel. This can also hinder our ability to critique or analyse sexuality socially, as if it seems not *cool* to say or think "no thanks" to any of the range of sexual behaviours we know about these days.

In this book, I am suggesting that it is not what we do, but how we feel about doing it that makes up a nutritious and satisfying sexual life. Do you wake up the next day thinking, oh no, what did I do, or wow, that was great, I feel so good? To understand how we feel, we need to consciously enquire into our sexuality, rather than treating it as something that "just happens". Readers might feel afraid that this would interfere with the spontaneity of sex, but I would argue just the opposite: by knowing ourselves, we are free to initiate and receive the kind of sexual contact we truly desire.

We live in a seemingly liberated sexual environment, with sexuality widely displayed. It is assumed that everyone (else) is having an amazing sex life with no problems, so individuals with difficulties can often feel inadequate and ashamed. Bringing these issues to light, understanding them individually and as a society, can help to alleviate the fear and anxieties often associated with discussing these subjects. It seems to be difficult for us socially to acknowledge explicitly the "shadow" side of our sexuality, such as sexual violence; therefore, it is more difficult for us to address. Perhaps by nature the shadow is hidden; however, this can cause more distress, as people feel embarrassed about their sexual difficulties, which compounds their problems.

LoveSex is divided into four sections: mind, brain, body, and emotion. Each section provides information and asks pertinent questions, drawing relationships between many different threads. With easy to read text, illustrations and diagrams, it describes the body and brain physiology of sexuality, and explores how what we believe and have experienced about sex informs our desires and sexual behaviour now. It identifies difficulties with current language and thinking and explores our implicit reproductive model of sex. It includes being conscious, respectful, and creative with our sexual energy—making love, not war. It honours the pleasure principle and the delights of intimacy that we can experience through our sexuality, in relationship with ourselves or with others.

Rather than offering answers, tips, or techniques about performance, this book asks many questions. You are invited to investigate your own answers by participating in a series of self-discovery exercises that have all been tried and tested through years of clinical practice and experiential trainings. Through these discoveries, you can clarify feelings, values, and beliefs about what turns you on and what turns you off—physically, emotionally, and mentally. You can explore who you want to be as a sexual being, how you want to express your sexuality, and who with. You can find out what kind of sexual diet suits you by becoming more mindful of your own sensual and sexual desires, tastes, and appetite.

We do not need to understand the workings of our bodies to have a good relationship with our sexuality, just as we do not need to understand the metabolism of digestion to eat well. However, most people who want to eat a nutritious diet do want to understand what our nutritional needs are, what foods provide proteins, carbohydrates, vitamins, minerals, etc. They want to know how to prepare and cook foods to maximise their benefits. We are surprisingly uneducated about ourselves sexually: what we need and how we "work". *LoveSex* offers an opportunity to learn more and to re-evaluate your sexual life. It aims to empower you, the reader, of any level of education or professional training, age, gender, or sexual orientation to consciously create a nutritious sexual life to be pleased with and proud of.

A new model for sexuality

As a concept to help us understand some of the different elements that are at play in any human sexual moment, we can expand on the body–mind paradigm and use the four distinctions of mind, body, brain, and emotion. We are familiar with the idea of the "head" or the mind being the part of us that is rational, our thinking part, and the body being the more irrational or emotive part of us. With regard to our sexuality, it can be helpful to distinguish what goes on in the *brain*, the back brain, which triggers our reactions, reflexes, and urges, from the *mind*, the front of our brain, as our rational thinking ability. We could think of this as the back of the skull and the forehead. In addition, we will consider the differences in our *body*, our physical sensations and sexual responses, from the feelings and *emotion* we may experience.

In reality, human experience is a relationship between all of these different aspects: our instincts, our physiology, feelings, and thoughts are affecting and being affected by each other and are all operating in unison, in a continual feedback loop. We cannot actually separate them or place them in any hierarchy, as all are equally important. Science and biology use the phrase "homeostasis" to describe how organisms rebalance in reactions to stimuli and responses. To understand human sexuality more deeply, it is useful to use the phrase "homeo-dynamic", coined by Rose (1999) to indicate the constant responses and interactions that happens in human being (Figure 1).

This new integrative model for sexuality incorporates research from neuroscience, complementary and alternative health therapies, and cognitive–behavioural therapy, along with psychotherapy and traditional eastern and western approaches to psychosexual therapy. It considers our sexuality with regard to these four different aspects, and also how they affect, and are affected by, each other. This model is a way of understanding what might be happening within an individual person, but humans do not exist in isolation; we are also social beings. We experience ourselves and behave in ways that are influenced by our society and culture. We are constantly in relationship, not only with ourselves (and all our internal body systems), but also with our external environment, other people, including our families, friends, and lovers. We need to consider all these factors and how they interact in relationship to our sexuality. Each section of this book explores all the dynamics of mind, body, brain, and emotion, individually and in depth, with a focus on sexuality. There is no order of preference, as all are interrelated and interdependent.

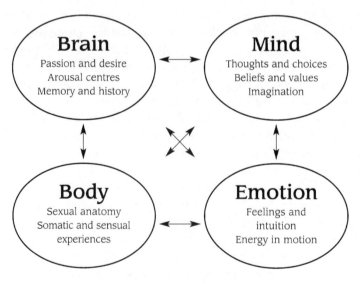

Figure 1. A homeodynamic model for sexuality.

• The *mind* can be thought of as the front brain and is home to our sexual values and beliefs. Humans have evolved with frontal lobes, which allow us to reflect on our reactions, to think, weigh up options, and make choices about our behaviour. We have imagination, the ability to anticipate and dream about the future. I am starting here as our beliefs and social cultures deeply inform our sexuality. Having an opportunity to question and re-evaluate our explicit and implicit belief systems allows us to identify issues for concern and to make more conscious choices. We can review what we believe, where we learnt these ideas and whether they still serve us. By analysing our unique history and our current social and cultural opinions about sexuality, we can contextualise our thinking. We can become clearer about what we really value about our sexuality and sexual relationships, about what suits us now as adults. We can gain some tools to change any outmoded ideas and sharpen our current belief system.

• Our *body* has a sexual anatomy and physiology that is little understood. By separating our reproductive and sexual functioning, we can learn more about sensuality and more fully understand and enjoy our physical sexual potential. For example, that ejaculation and orgasm are distinguishable, and that both men and women are capable of multiple orgasms (Chia & Abrams, 2002a,b, Chia & Carlton Abrams, 2005). Sexual arousal on a physical level is sensual arousal, stimulation of the senses. Some sights, sounds, tastes, smells, touch, and ways of being touched turn us on, and others turn us off. We can find out more about ourselves sexually by exploring sensuality in depth, including all the various body systems, as well as our genitals, that are involved in sexual arousal. This is particularly useful where there are obstacles to sexual arousal, such as erectile difficulties, lack of clitoral arousal, or lack of vaginal lubrication. We can develop a more intimate connection to our own body and thus discover and become more conscious about what arouses pleasure and what does not; a subjective experience of feeling sexual rather than what we look like to others.

• The back *brain* triggers our reflexive survival abilities, such as the adrenaline rush of fight and flight or our desires and urges for sex and food. It is home to our limbic system: the name given to a cluster of organs in the brain, which are activated when we react to any stimulus to our system. It includes our memory centres, which are used to process reactions by using our knowledge, our history, to evaluate responses in any given moment. Understanding the neurochemistry of sexual arousal allows for a wider view of our imperatives for being sexual and the impact of sexual trauma. We can see passion and desire as impulsive reactions from our back brain, as distinct from the thinking abilities of our frontal lobes, our mind. We can explore issues concerning sexual desire to help clarify our own sexual identity: who we are attracted to, what behaviours we wish to express with them, and also when, how, and why. We can discover more about our "reactivity" and the triggers which turn arousal on, or turn it off, and how this links with our personal history. Such explorations are useful to address sexual difficulties which affect both arousal and desire, like rapid or delayed ejaculation, orgasm difficulties, unconscious tightening of vaginal or anal muscles, or where there is pain during intercourse.

• The *emotions* and feelings are our experience of the energy that is set in motion through the body by the triggers that have stimulated any of the above. A feeling can be an emotion like love, grief, fear, or anger, or it can be physical sensations, such as feeling hot or cold, tightness in the stomach, or a headache. A feeling might be a hunch, a guess, or maybe a thought. Sometimes, it is a combination of all of these. We can explore the myriad feelings and emotions that surround human sexuality and their impact on our experience of sexuality. A focus on social issues provides a wider context for some of the sexual issues people contend with. This includes sexual shame, addiction and compulsivity, and the impact of sexual violence. Many people have concerns about seeking sexual relationships or sustaining current relationships. Relationship issues are discussed, such as communication skills, managing difference, and conflict. Sexual health is explored in terms of physical, emotional, mental, and spiritual well-being.

In reality, all sections or elements are triggering and responding to all the others, all the time. There is a constant dialogue and communication between our brain, our body systems and body organs, and back again, all in nano-seconds. Our thinking, brain chemistry, and physiology are constantly online, reacting and responding, creating a circular and interacting flow. Every reaction in our brain causes physiological changes, which in turn trigger emotions and thoughts, which, again, trigger more reactions. This could be seen as a circle, as a circuit of arousal that can be switched on or be broken, and be switched off. By drawing all these aspects together, how they affect and are affected by each other, we can consider the preciousness and fragilities of our lived human experiences of sexuality, and begin to develop a new framework and model for sexual self-esteem. Given the knowledge and confidence of this self-esteem, we can more consciously create a model for psychosexual health, individually and socially.

Introduction to sexploration exercises

Getting started

The sexploration exercises are a crucial aspect of this book and this model: rather than telling you what to think or believe, what you should be doing or wanting to do, *LoveSex* invites you to find out for yourself. Through doing these exercises, you can learn about yourself, physically, mentally, and emotionally, which can help you to identify and integrate a sexual self-esteem.

How you use this book may depend on why it interests you. Those I have most often worked with have a general curiosity about sexuality, are individuals or couples with a specific sexual difficulty, are survivors of sexual abuse, or are professional therapists or students working with clients' sexual issues. Feel free to skip any sections in this introduction that do not feel relevant for you.

The exercises are set within the format of the homeodynamic for sexuality. In each of the sections of *mind, body, brain,* and *emotion* there are several chapters, each of which provides information and asks questions. At the end of each chapter is an exercise presented in a box for you to explore what you think or feel. They do follow a flow, but you can choose to start or focus where you like. You might like to consider each exercise as it is presented, or you might prefer to read each section and then go back over the exercises. There is a review of each section. You might prefer to read the whole book and then consider if and which exercises appeal to you. You could allow your "work" with these exercises to mirror a new approach to your sexuality by noticing the quality of how you set about this, rather than the quantity of how much you get done.

Exercise   A journal for your journey

You may want to make or buy yourself a special journal to write about the exercises in this book. Choose something that represents your sexuality. It may be about the cover, a picture, the colour or design. It may be about the paper inside, whether it has a lock or not or about how much it costs.

You may prefer to express yourself through art, music or sculpture. Collect or buy the art and crafts materials you may want to use.

When you have your journal or materials, reflect on why you have chosen what you have, and how it represents your sexuality.

Through my years of work with numerous different people, I am aware that this work can have a profound impact, sometimes more than we expect. I am not referring in particular to extremes such as repressed memories, though this can happen, just that consciously exploring our sexuality is a powerful and vulnerable aspect of our humanity, which culturally we tend to keep hidden and shrouded in shame. Gentle explorations can and often do trigger uncomfortable feelings. Therefore, a crucial element is to first create a safe space.

Exercise   Create a safe sexploration space

Identify a room or physical space where you feel private, comfortable, warm, relaxed, undisturbed, and whatever else is important to you. Think about the words privacy and secrecy; what do they mean to you, how are they different and how similar. Create a safe private space for yourself, the physical space, the lighting and ambience. Do you like candles or aromas? Notice what you like and want, and what you do not want.

Create a safe emotional space, too. Identify a nice space for yourself where you can do this work at your own pace, where you feel comfortable and relaxed. It can be useful to have some "anchors", such as using a time limit, especially if you know a particular exercise might feel difficult. If you find an exercise becoming difficult emotionally, be kind and gentle with yourself. Take a pause; decide if you want to continue now or maybe later, when you have had time to consider what is difficult or why.

It can be helpful to get support; tell a friend or therapist what you are doing and how you are feeling, maybe ask them to be with you while you do a specific exercise, or ask if you can speak to them afterwards about it. This can help create a "container" for strong emotions, just knowing someone else is there to care for and support you.

After each exercise, spend some time thinking and reflecting on your thoughts and feelings. Write, draw, or phone a friend, whatever feels right to you.

A note for survivors of sexual violence

If you have experienced sexual violence as an adult, or childhood sexual abuse, the impact of doing this work might be more profound, so issues of self-care are even more important. Recovery and reclaiming a sense of sexual self-esteem might require several stages, depending on each person's unique needs. Psychotherapeutic support is invaluable for the "relational" aspects of betrayal and violation, and for the confusing and complex physical and sexual *survival* responses that people often experience during abuse. By learning more about your own "psychosexual processes" through these exercises, you can identify and remedy disruptions to your sexual ease. It might be helpful to do this work within a therapeutic relationship or with the support of friends, someone you feel safe with, to share any thoughts and feelings that might be evoked during your explorations. Bodywork and a variety of complementary health therapies and spiritual practices can also help. Sexual healing can help people to move through to thriving once again, to reclaiming a sense of sexual joy and playfulness, and an enjoyment of intimacy and sharing, sexual love and pleasure.

One legacy of sexual violence is that strong feelings can be easily triggered; we can feel scared, confused, or enraged if old traumas are re-stimulated. Through these exercises, you can discover where you may still have disharmony due to your past. Memories will affect *brain* responses to stimuli. Physical sensations in your *body* or certain *emotions* might trigger you back into trauma. What goes on in your *mind* might cause distress. Usually, a combination of all of these can occur. It is, therefore, useful to know how to check in with your arousal process, to understand a bit more about what is happening and learn to be able to "apply the brakes", take some time to relax, and soothe yourself. Any "trigger" will cause automatic scanning of our memory centres; there may be a re-stimulation of any "horrible history" where arousal was overwhelming. Learning to understand and manage our responses to our reflexes brings a reclaiming of our bodies.

First, I recommend that you create your safe space, as outlined above. Another idea is of creating anchors to support therapeutic work. Choose something or someone that you associate with a feeling of safety, relief, and well-being, physically and emotionally. For example, a grandparent, a favourite pet, a special object, a hobby, or a place. The next exercise is important for anyone doing this work. It was developed by Rothschild (2000), particularly for working safely with recovery from trauma. If we become flooded by feelings, stress hormones activate the sympathetic nervous system. This can send us into overdrive, causing "hyper arousal": an increase in heartbeat, rapid breathing, and muscle tension. We can feel "frozen", unable to move or speak. Our thinking process is impaired and we might feel exposed and at risk.

Any reader should read this exercise through and practise "applying the brakes" before driving this car, this sexploration. It can then be used throughout, or whenever the need arises. If you know or think you have trauma in your history, it is useful to practise until you can contain your anxieties, emotions, and body sensations *at will*.

Exercise   Applying the brakes

It takes longer to bring the *relaxing* part of the nervous system back on line than for the *arousal* to trigger—you need to give it time. You will not be able to think clearly to choose the next step until you calm your body.

You can start exploring this now. Just the fact of reading these pages probably means that the curiosity circuit in your brain has fired, causing an arousal of energy in your body. Put your hands over your heart area and notice your heartbeat. And breathe—if you are holding your breath!

As you are doing the exercises, pay attention to your heartbeat and breath, as they indicate levels of physiological arousal, which happens when we feel joy or pleasure, too. If you are experiencing difficult or intense feelings, panic, or anxiety, you need to "apply the brakes".

It helps to sit down, put your feet on the ground, and take some deep breaths. Just keep focusing on breathing in and out, long slow out-breaths. You will see how this slowing down can soothe how you feel. It can take some practice. You could imagine you are blowing the breath out through a straw.

Narrowing your focus to the here and now helps to calm also. Notice your body sensations. Look around the room and notice what you see. Maybe say words aloud. Remind yourself you are in your safe space. Remember your anchor(s). Just keep focusing on your breathing; allow the breath in and slowly out, releasing any tension you are holding, particularly in your jaw, neck, or shoulders.

Notice your thoughts—are they calming and soothing? If not, consider why you are saying mean things to yourself and try to be more kind. When you are ready, go back to the previous exercise and reconsider your Safe Space; make any alterations you might need. If necessary, it can be useful to consider this exercise again before you start each new chapter of the book.

A note on psychosexual difficulties

There are a wide range of psychosexual issues that challenge individuals and couples, and these are addressed throughout this book. Although the exercises might help, other specific support might be needed. There are many website references at the end of this book. Two common sexual issues for which people seek help are about a lack of, or impaired, sexual interest, and physical difficulties with sexual arousal. It is useful to distinguish between these two, although they are often related and can exacerbate each other.

It is useful to know whether there is a lack of arousal because there is no desire to be sexual, for example, with a specific person, or to partake in specific sexual activities. If there is desire but there are difficulties with physical sexual arousal, this can, in time, lead to a lack of desire, because wanting to be sexual but not being able to can bring feelings of distress and/or pressures about developing or sustaining relationships. A good starting point for understanding the root causes of sexual difficulties is to ask some questions to clarify what helps or hinders the situation and to uncover more about the meaning for the individual. Physical issues will be happening within a framework of beliefs and values, and feelings and emotions, so it is also worth exploring the exercises in those chapters.

- If there is a complete lack of sexual desire, is it connected to other physical or psychological symptoms? Is it being affected by the side effects of medication or hormonal changes due to menopause or aging? If not, what are the circumstances in which desire is more present or less available? Are there any sexual daydreams or interest in masturbation? Is there a "relationship issue", such as bereavement, fertility issues, or conflict in the relationship?

- If there are difficulties with genital erections, is this total or partial? When or during which activities does the situation improve or what makes it worse? Does the arousal begin but is not sustained?

- Some women experience an involuntary tightening of the vagina muscles, which hinders penetration. This difficulty can also affect the anal muscles. There may be pain during penetration. Does this always happen, and if not, which situations or scenarios make it better or worse? Is there adequate arousal and lubrication before attempting penetration? Does this happen during masturbation or only during sex with a partner?

- Any of the above issues may also influence experiences of orgasm and/or ejaculation, so are worthy of the same questions about circumstances and about the quality and levels of arousal. If ejaculation is experienced as happening prematurely, we could ask, too soon for what? Is it pleasurable when it does occur? At what stage of arousal or sexual behaviour does ejaculation happen, is there anything that helps to delay it or which makes it worse? Does this also happen during masturbation, or only with a partner?

While this book focuses on the links between our body, mind, and emotions, it is important to understand or discover whether there is a medical or organic cause for a sexual difficulty, as this will influence the way forward. For example, if a man has no morning erection, or if there are no circumstances in which the person feels desire or is able to become sexually aroused, a medical investigation by either a GP or a doctor at a sexual health clinic might help identify why. It is a good idea to get a check-up about physical sexual difficulties, as they can sometimes be indications of other health problems, such as diabetes or heart conditions. Schnarch (1998) and Irwin (2002) both provide lists of the health conditions that have an impact on sexual functioning, and also of the many medications that have side effects that can affect sexual desire and/or arousal.

Some suffer through the hormonal rollercoaster of the menopause, or with other issues due to aging. People might have physical impairments or be suffering from chronic or long-term illness. There can sometimes be physical difficulties due to injuries sustained during the birthing process, from accidents, or through sexual violence. There might also be physical abnormality in the size or shape of the genitals, making some sexual behaviour difficult or impossible. For these circumstances, there are sex aids to support as fulfilling a sex life as possible. (For examples, see www.spokz.co.uk; www.ableize.com; www.disabilities-r-us.com/sexuality; www.mypleasure.com.) These can be discussed with a psychosexual therapist or through investigation of dedicated websites. It is often useful also to consider counselling to address any psychological issues associated with these difficulties and/or to support incorporating the use of sex aids into a person or couple's sexual life. All of the above issues might require new ways of thinking about sex and new ways of behaving sexually to incorporate the physical needs of individuals.

A note for professional therapists or students

Psychosexual therapy is educational, behavioural, and psychotherapeutic. The text provides the educational material and the exercises a way of investigating the issues for the individual. Working psychotherapeutically means working within the therapeutic relationship to explore the responses to the exercises and what they mean to the individual.

The guidelines as recommended above will adequately address any concerns for counsellors or therapists wishing to use these exercises with clients. Within this model, it is most helpful if professionals do any exercise themselves before recommending it to clients. This provides more than a theoretical approach to the work; it gives a deeper understanding of each exercise, how it may affect a client, and when it might be useful or not. I strongly recommend that you first read the exercise "Applying the brakes" and familiarise yourself with the signs of traumatic re-stimulation, so that you may help clients work safely around psychosexual issues. You might wish also to read Herman's (1993) work on traumatic transference. Another tool suggested by Hawton (1985) for understanding any sexual issues is to consider:

- predisposing factors: what issues might have happened in someone's childhood, in their history;
- precipitating factors: what has triggered them to seek help now? This can be a source of support in their recovery, as it often is part of the motivation to change;
- maintaining factors: can indicate what might get in the way of change; what are the behaviours or attitudes that might have to be given up, in order to allow change to happen.

Primarily, the professional therapist will be working within the remit of the therapeutic relationship. Ideas to use certain exercises will come through that perspective. It is always advisable to go slowly, make suggestions, and work therapeutically with the client's response: is it an exercise they feel keen to try or not? The focus is on the *how*, the quality, not *how much, how fast*, an important distinction as a mirror for sexuality. For some clients, the work is to find their "no" before they can find their "yes". Not wanting to do an exercise, and the therapist not only allowing that, but encouraging and supporting their choice, *is* the therapeutic work.

If in doubt about psychosexual work, you could always refer on to an experienced and qualified integrative psychosexual therapist, who will have undergone a minimum of two years intense training and exploration of many of the ideas discussed in this book (see Centre for Psychosexual Health; College of Sexual and Relationship Therapists; UK Association of Humanistic Psychology Practitioners). This will usually have included a personal experience of all the exercises, leading to reflection and discussion of the personal and professional implications of this work. It will have included experience of working with real client issues, in-depth supervision on therapeutic practice, and an understanding of transferential and countertransferential issues common in working with sexual issues. This results in an expertise and skilfulness in recommending and working with the exercises in this book, understanding the usefulness, appropriateness, and safety issues of any particular exercise.

Finally . . .

Overall, this series of sexploration exercises is about relationships; our relationship to our own bodies and our own sexuality, to our own sexual beliefs and behaviours. This informs us, and so allows a more conscious choice about the sexual relationships we engage in. Many exercises in this book can be done by couples, together or alone, and then shared or discussed together or with friends, or as part of individual or couple therapy.

What is at the heart of these exercises is a model for psychosexual health, where we can feel proud about our sexuality and have a nutritious and healthy sexual self-esteem. This includes mental, physical, social, and emotional aspects of sexuality. When we, as individuals and as a society, have a sex-affirmative attitude, which honours our sexual capacity and abilities, we can see our human sexual potential as a life force that offers love, creativity, and pleasure; all vital aspects of being human. These exercises are an opportunity to update our sexual knowledge, both generally and personally, and to evaluate our relationship to our sexuality.

PART I

MIND: THOUGHTS AND CHOICES

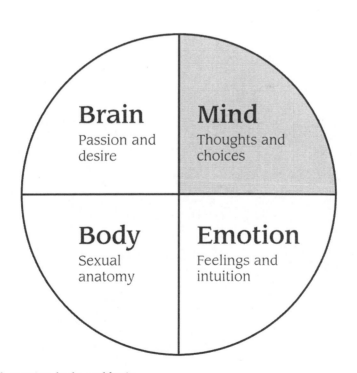

Mind, emotion, body, and brain.

The mind

This exploration into sexuality begins by evaluating our thinking and beliefs so we can become more mindful, more conscious as individuals and as a society. To answer questions about what is a healthy sexual appetite or healthy sexual diet, we will address the interplay between our biological urges and our social conditioning, our bodies and our feelings. A main principle of this book is relationships; how all these facets interrelate with one another. But first let us separate some of the parts. By reviewing some evolutionary developments in humans, we can re-evaluate our thinking about sex and sexuality, including our beliefs and values, sex education, sexual orientation, sexual health, relationships, and the pleasure principle.

An exciting awareness, developed from studies in psychotherapy and neuroscience, is the idea of there being different evolutionary aspects to the human brain (Panksepp, 1998; Sunderland, 2007). Like mammals, we have an area of the brain devoted to survival reactions such as fight and flight. These reflexes are triggered from an area of the brain called the limbic system, or the "emotional brain". They include our instinctual defensive reactions, programmed from when humans shared the planet with sabre-toothed tigers. If in danger, we needed a quick-fire response. In this book, this *reactive* aspect of humans will be called the brain, and will be discussed in detail in the next section.

Humans have also developed frontal lobes in our brain, which give us the capacity to think, to reflect on our feelings and urges. For example, we might feel our heart beat faster if we saw a tiger, a reaction triggered by the instinctual brain. This would begin to slow down once the frontal lobes had processed various factors, thought about it, and reminded us that we are not in danger if, for example, we are in a zoo. All of this will have happened in nano-seconds. We will distinguish this *reflective* aspect of the brain from the reactive areas, by calling it the mind, the subject of this section.

This ability to reflect gives us a consciousness and allows us to choose, and decide on, our behaviour. We make lots of decisions every day, mediating between how we feel, our urges, and what we do, how we act. We might not feel like getting up for work on a cold morning, but we do; we might feel like crying or shouting at someone, but decide, for various reasons, not to. We might feel a sexual urge, but be aware that it is not an appropriate time or place to act on that desire. This is an important distinction for psychosexual work, since our sexual arousal process is a reflexive reaction from the instinctual brain. There are many aspects of the reflective mind, explored and discussed in this section, which influence how we think and feel about sex and sexuality and how we behave sexually.

Exercise   First thoughts

What do you *think* about sex? Write down the first three words that come to mind when you think about sex and sexuality. Try to catch, not censor, your very first thoughts, your mind talk.

Sex:

1.

2.

3.

Sexuality:

1.

2.

3.

Inner dialogue

By separating the reflexive reactions in the brain from the thinking aspects of the frontal lobes, we can explore how our beliefs inform our thinking, how our thinking influences our feelings, and how they, in turn, influence our behaviour, whether we are conscious of this or not. By being more conscious about our mind-talk, our internal dialogue, we become clearer about what we do actually think and why we believe what we do. By evaluating and analysing the quality of our inner dialogue, we can see whether it is, in fact, a bullying voice, constantly moaning and telling us off, or an inner wise voice, gently questioning us, guiding us, helping us to see our mistakes and giving advice about how to improve things for next time. For example, if we ask for something we want but are rejected, do we tell ourselves that we were stupid for wanting that thing in the first place or crazy for believing we deserved it, or do we feel our disappointment, re-evaluate whether we do actually still want this thing, and if we do, maybe go somewhere else to ask for it? We will discuss in more detail in the "Emotion" section how child developmental phases are the building blocks of healthy self-esteem, and how our own specific histories will have supported or damaged our perceptions and abilities as adults.

A useful model to understand this further is that of ego states, developed by Berne (1961). The idea is that we have three aspects to our personality: parent, child, and adult. The parent includes conditioning and socialisation: beliefs about what we *should* do. The child is seen to include our natural spontaneous reactions: emotions, feelings, needs, and desires, and is related to our past, our childhood. The adult aspect is seen as the part of us capable of making informed choices: we are able to process the information from our parent and child part, think and reflect, and make decisions about our behaviour.

The parent part can have two aspects: nurturing, which is educative, caring, supportive, and helpful, or controlling, which is critical, bullying, and judgemental. Children who grow up in nurturing environments, with their basic needs met, will develop a strong "free child", who loves to play, feels free to be a child, but essentially will also respect boundaries and co-operate with the adults in their lives. Children who do not will become "wounded" and their child part can become "withdrawn"—passive, conformist, and manipulative—in

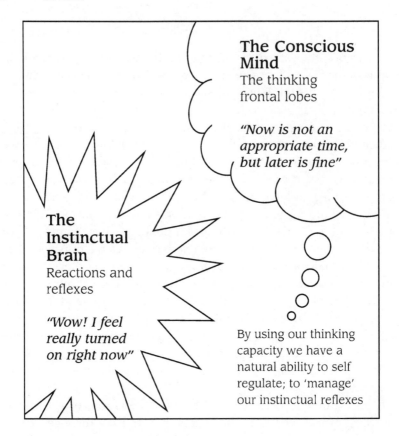

Figure 2.   Two aspects of the human brain.

order to get their needs met. Alternatively, they can become "rebellious"—angry, fighting, and anti-authoritarian, with a strongly internalised "controlling parent".

How we dialogue internally between the reactive and reflective aspects within ourselves will also be mirrored in our interactions with others. If we have a strong inner critic, we will often be quite critical of others, and probably not have the good negotiation and communication skills vital for maintaining sexual relationships. The role of assertiveness includes self-awareness and an ability to manage our feelings. We need to know what we feel and think, before we can communicate and negotiate with others.

A sense of empowerment and inner self-esteem can come from being more mindful; choosing our beliefs, accepting our feelings as reactions and responses, and then using our mind to reflect, evaluate, and then choose, as much as possible, how we want to behave. The quality of our inner dialogue will be explored more in depth later in the "Emotion" section, where we will see that a critical inner voice is often a greater source of distress to us than our emotions: what we tell ourselves about what we are feeling and whether it is acceptable to have such feelings causing more anguish than the emotion itself.

Exercise   Inner critic

Take five minutes to think about your "mind talk" in a general sense. Notice your inner dialogue and how it is you talk to yourself. What sort of words do you use; are they kind or critical? What about the tone of your words? Say some common phrases that you use out loud, what is it like to hear them? Evaluate whether you think the quality of your self-reflection is useful, or bullying and critical.

Choose one thing you criticise yourself about sexually and see whether there could be a different phrase or comment, or way of thinking about it, that could actually help you to change something.

Beliefs

We have many social and cultural values and belief systems about human sexuality, which are historically steeped in shame and taboos. These taboos are reflected in the fact that many of our swearwords have a sexual nature. The social sentiment of many of the words used shows our disgust and social shame. References to male genitalia, such as calling someone a prick or dickhead, imply a somewhat affectionately viewed stupidity, but references to female genitalia imply serious contempt.

What we believe and value about human sexuality, both socially and individually, will inform our experiences and expressions of our sexuality. We rarely take time to consider these issues and to evaluate what are biological imperatives and what are social constructs. We rarely think about our sexual values: what is really valuable to us individually about our sexual desires, beliefs, and how we choose to express ourselves and act sexually.

There are many social and relational elements to human sexuality: as well as our physiological urges, emotions, and psychology, there is a desire for pleasure. Despite our cultural taboos about sex and sexuality, we humans like and express our sexuality in many ways, from how we dress to flirting, dancing, and engaging in sexual acts, alone or with other people. Some people divert their sexual energy into spiritual practices or into creative acts such as painting or dancing. We do not have to channel our sexual energy into sexual acts or sexual reproduction.

Our social and cultural beliefs and values are very varied and often emotionally charged. We have religious beliefs and laws about sexual behaviour that predominantly espouse a reproductive model of sex—that real sex *is* heterosexual intercourse. Many people define loss of virginity by having experienced heterosexual intercourse, and, in slang, "doing it" means having penetration. Until 2003, the crime of rape was defined solely as non-consensual penis-to-vagina penetration. It now includes any type of non-consensual penetration to any orifice (Office of Public Sector Information, 2003).

Most children's first introduction to the world of human sexuality is about reproduction; about something that adults do to make babies. We talk about sexual relationships in marriages or couples cohabiting as a unit to raise children together, as a family. Through our highly sexualised media, we are also learning that many adults engage in a variety of other sexual behaviours and encounters. In recent years, sex education in schools has focused on having sex or not having sex; if you do have sex you should use contraception and/or have safer sex by using a condom, which again supports the belief that sex is sexual intercourse.

We rarely think about what we believe, where we got our beliefs from, and how they influence us. This leads us to believe that others share our beliefs and that they are facts, rather than opinions. Our focus on sex as something we do, rather than being sexual as something that we are, encourages us to think about the quantity of our sex life, not the quality of our sexual expression.

We talk little about feeling sexual or the emotional and relational reasons for sexual desire, or about the fact that it is usually an "other" that we want to be sexual with. It is important to reflect on what we were taught about sex and sexuality and what we believe now, because it will be unconsciously, if not consciously, influencing our expressions of our sexuality, including our sexual behaviour.

Exercise   Sexual beliefs

Write down something/s that you *believe* about the following; go with your first thoughts.

My sexuality

Women and sex

Men and sex

Sexual identity

Sexual relationships

Review what you have written; reflect on the words or phrases. Does anything surprise you? Write about how you feel about what you have written.

Sexual language

How we think about sexuality is also influenced by language: by the language we were taught as children and what words and concepts we use culturally. Even though sex seems to be everywhere in our culture, we are still surprisingly embarrassed and uneducated, not at ease with acknowledging and discussing this aspect of our humanity.

Our first introduction to the word sex is probably in response to us asking where babies come from. School sex education starts with the biology of reproduction: about grown-ups "making love"; about a man and a woman having sexual intercourse. With children, we reflect our discomfort with sex by using euphemisms for sexualised body parts and sexual behaviours. We have words that are used interchangeably but mean different things to different people. For example, the word *sex* may be used to mean gender, a sexual act, or sexuality. The word *sexuality* is often used to refer to non-heterosexual matters, such as working with sexual minorities. The phrase *sexual health* usually refers to sexually transmitted infections. It can be useful to think about your use of language for all sexualised body parts and sexual activities: what are the technical terms and what are your preferred words? It can be difficult to discuss sexual matters when we do not have a language we feel comfortable with.

We implicitly teach our children that sex is for procreation; that sex is something that we *do*—we have sex, we make love *to* someone. Thinking about "our sexuality" allows us to see it as an expression of ourselves and our personality, as something that we *are*. It is important to be able to separate our sexual feelings and our sexual behaviour, to recognise that feelings come from the reactive brain and choices about our behaviour emanate from our mind. Seeing our sexuality as something we can express in many more ways than sexual intercourse allows us to explore our sexual desires and attractions in a new way.

Exercise   Sexual knowledge

Explore the following statements:

What I learnt about sex as a child was . . .

What I learnt about sex as a teenager was . . .

What I have learnt about sex as an adult is . . .

Reflect on what you've written and then write:

What I want to know about sex is . . .

Sexual culture

In Britain, we live in a highly sexualised culture where images are widely displayed in our media and sex is referred to and alluded to often. We are also still very shame-bound as a culture, with a pervasive lack of ease about our sexuality. One reaction to this background, and perhaps an attempt to overcome it, is a new cultural shamelessness, a notion that really liberated people, with no sexual hang-ups, will have no boundaries, will do anything with anyone, anywhere. It is very different for people to consciously choose as expressive a sexual life as they want and people feeling ashamed or frigid for not wanting to engage in certain sexual behaviours.

Many girls and boys in Britain who have sexual intercourse under the age of sixteen cite alcohol, pornography, and peer pressure as their main reason for doing so, and the majority expressed subsequent regret (Redgrave & Limmer, 2005). Comparative studies show a different picture in the Netherlands, where sex education focuses more on gender issues, intimacy, and taking responsibility. Boys in Britain are four times more likely to cite peer pressure as a reason for having first sex, while Dutch boys are more than five times more likely to cite love and commitment than UK boys (Family Education Trust, 2003).

Many teenagers now report getting their primary information about sex from Internet pornography and taking these unrealistic impressions as "normal" and judging non-cosmetically enhanced breasts and/or genitals as disgusting. Sixty-one per cent cite concerns about the appearance of their own genitals and forty per cent of males (wrongly) believe their penises are smaller than average. Sixty per cent say that pornography has an impact on their sex lives, with many reporting unsafe sexual practices (Richardson, 2010).

How realistic are our current beliefs and images about looking, and therefore being, sexy? What impact does all this have on our experience of our sexuality, our sexual practices, and our sexual self-esteem? A chronic lack of self-esteem about body image is expressed by both men and women (Swami & Furnham, 2008), in comparison to the images of ultra-thin celebrities and airbrushed glamour models. In a recent survey of fourteen- to seventeen-year-olds, twenty-seven per cent of boys reported being unhappy with their penises and forty-five per cent of girls were unhappy with their breasts. There has been a 465% increase in cosmetic surgery in the past ten years (Dines, 2010), and a 300% increase in labia surgery in the past five years (Richardson, 2009). A recent study into the largely unregulated industry says the risks include permanent scarring, infections, bleeding, and irritation (Cardozo, 2011). There is also a risk of increased or decreased sensitivity if nerves get caught in the operation, which, given our general lack of knowledge about the true extent of the clitoral system, is a real possibility.

Exercise   Who taught you?

Think about what you have written about in the exercise 'Sexual knowledge' above and consider more explicitly who helped to inform you about sex and sexuality.

What I learnt from my parents or carers . . .

What I learnt from school and/or religion . . .

What I learnt from my siblings or peer group . . .

What I have learnt from my own experience . . .

Write, think, or draw about what you have written. Has anything surprised you? Contemplate and re-evaluate. Which of your beliefs feel right for you now? Are some outmoded? Identify one *belief* you want to change and what you want to change it to.

Sex and reproduction

The distinction between our sexual and reproductive functioning is not made explicit. Yes, humans do reproduce through having sexual intercourse, but humans do not have sex just to reproduce. Female humans are potentially sexually potent all their adult lives, despite being physiologically fertile for an amazingly short time. During each monthly menstrual cycle, women are "infertile" except for a few days around ovulation, when they have a ripened egg that could be fertilised. So, there are only a few days in each month when a woman *could* conceive (Women's Health, 2012). However, females are sexually functional during the times when they are fertile and when they are not, including after the menopause. Males are physiologically fertile most of their adult life and can also experience sexual pleasure without ejaculating sperm. When ejaculation and orgasm are distinguished, for example, we can see that both men and women are capable of multiple orgasms. This will all be discussed more fully in the section titled "Body".

By focusing on sex as an act, rather than sexuality as something that is an innate part of us that we want to express, we miss out on connecting with our sexual energy, our fire, and our creative forces. *Doing* sex rather than *being* sexual misses out on the subtleties and nuances of relationship and encourages us to ignore the impact and any consequences. As with all energy on this planet, our sexual energy is something we could think about more ecologically.

Humans frequently engage in sexual intercourse when conception is not even possible, since adult women are not fertile for most of their adult life. There is also a huge repertoire of sexual behaviours other than intercourse that people engage in, including kissing, cuddling, playing, masturbating yourself or another, oral and anal sex (Masters, Johnson, & Kolodny, 1994). A quick analysis of any average 100 sexual acts on any one day shows us that our biological reproductive chances are surprisingly low. Since the 1950s, researchers have claimed that probably only one in ten sexual acts was heterosexual intercourse (Hite, 1976; Kinsey, Wardell, & Martin, 1948, 1953). This would leave ten sexual acts that could result in a conception. In 2007–2008, government statistics say seventy-five per cent of women in Great Britain use contraception (National Statistics Online, 2011), lowering the odds to two and a half chances of a conception from any average 100 sexual acts. Bearing in mind that women could be in the infertile phase of a monthly cycle, pregnant or menopausal, and current rates of infertility, it is actually amazing we get pregnant at all.

And yet, despite our array of contraception, there are thousands of conceptions, many unplanned and many unwanted. There were 189,100 abortions carried out in England and Wales in 2009, mostly funded by the NHS (Department of Health, 2009). Ninety-one per cent were carried out at less than thirteen weeks gestation and seventy-five per cent at less than ten weeks. There is also "emergency contraception", which can be used to help prevent an unwanted pregnancy up to five days after sex. This can include the "morning after pill" or having an intrauterine device (IUD) fitted. This is classified as "medical abortions", which account for forty per cent of the total.

Marie Stopes opened Britain's first birth control clinic in 1921. Although this required a societal acceptance of sex as playing more than a procreative role in people's lives, there is still an implicit assumption in "Family Planning" that sex is "intromission: the ejaculation of semen into the vagina". Data from the Health Protection Agency (2009) and The Sexual Health Charity FPA show the range and use of current contraception (used to prevent conception) and contragestions (used to prevent implantation). The most commonly used contraceptives are the pill (thirty-five to forty-three per cent) and the male condom (thirty to thirty-six per cent), (Department of Health, 2009; Family Planning Association, 2007). In 2008–2009, seventy-five per cent of women under fifty were using at least one method of contraception (Office for National Statistics, 2011):

- 25%—the contraceptive pill;
- 25%—the male condom;
- 17%—sterilisation;
- 8%—IUD / IUS;
- 3%—hormonal injection;

- 25% were not currently using a method of contraception, half of whom were not engaged in a sexual relationship with someone of the opposite sex.

Hormonal contraceptives include the combined pill, the contraceptive patch, and the new vaginal ring (Nuvaing), all of which combine oestrogen and progesterone.

- The combined pill includes twenty-seven types of oral medication.
- The contraceptive vaginal ring is a soft, plastic ring about four millimetres thick, and five and a half centimetres in diameter, which goes into the vagina.
- The contraceptive patch is placed on the arm.
- They all work by stopping ovulation, thickening the mucus around the cervix, and making the lining of the womb thinner, so that a fertilised egg would not be able to implant. They have an effectiveness rate of ninety-nine per cent.

The mini pill, contraceptive injections, and implants all contain progesterone only.

- The mini pill works because the progesterone thickens the mucus around the cervix, and makes the lining of the womb thinner so that a fertilised egg would not be able to implant. In some women, it stops ovulation and has the advantage of being able to be used when breastfeeding.
- The most commonly used contraceptive injection in Britain is Depo-Provera, where one injection lasts for twelve weeks. The contraceptive implant is a small, flexible rod, which is put under the skin in your upper arm, where it releases progesterone. Like the mini pill, it can be ninety-nine per cent effective.
- The intrauterine device (IUD) is sometimes called the "coil". It is a small T-shaped piece of plastic and copper that is inserted into the vagina, through the cervix, and into the uterus. The intrauterine system (IUS) is similar, except that it contains hormones. Both are claimed to be ninety-eight per cent effective in preventing pregnancy for five years or more and both can have side effects including breast tenderness, irregular or heavy bleeding.

Barrier methods include the male and female condoms, diaphragms and caps with spermicide, and the contraceptive sponge.

- Condoms are number one for protection against sexually transmitted infections (STIs) and are between ninety-five and ninety-eight per cent effective in preventing pregnancy, if used correctly: every time you have sex, put on before the penis touches or rubs against the vagina or anus. They are free in many places and have no side effects. They are the only method that a man can use to control his own fertility and make sure that he does not become a father before he is ready.
- Diaphragms and caps are dome-shaped and fit into the vagina and over the cervix. They must be fitted to ensure the correct size is used. They must both be used with spermicide and can then be ninety-two to ninety-six per cent effective.
- The contraceptive sponge also fits into the vagina and over the cervix and contains spermicide. It can be seventy-seven to ninety-one per cent effective in preventing pregnancy when used correctly.
- The most commonly used spermicide is Nonoxynol-9 (N-9); it is in contraceptive foams, creams, suppositories, and films. It disrupts the outer barrier of sperm and other cells and has been shown to be quite effective at killing many STI pathogens, including HIV, herpes, chlamydia, and gonorrhoea. It can be problematic when used frequently or in high doses, as it can cause inflammation or damage cells in the vagina and cervix, which might render a woman more susceptible to STIs.

Sterilisation is intended as a permanent form of contraception that will prevent pregnancy for ever. Surgery can be done to reverse it, but is not always successful. Both men and women can be sterilised. Women can have an operation to cut or block their fallopian tubes. This means that eggs will never be able to reach the womb. Men can have the tubes that carry the sperm cut so that they do not produce sperm when they ejaculate (this is called a vasectomy).

Natural family planning is when a woman avoids unprotected intercourse during the fertile phase of her monthly cycle. Every woman is different and needs to learn to observe and understand her "basic infertile pattern" (which will be explained later), and then also the changes in her body temperature and cervical fluids that occur to indicate fertility during each cycle. (The fertile cycle is explained in more depth in the section titled "Body".) Using our knowledge about women's fertility cycles has really only caught our attention since the increased awareness of infertility. Rather than the belief that women can get pregnant at any time, it has become evident that there is actually only a brief window of opportunity. Fertility monitoring devices such as ovulation tests have been developed using the indicators outlined above. The fertility awareness method (FAM) includes the above indicators of fertility, but also involves monitoring the cervical variations during the month and other subjective changes, and using barrier methods if intercourse is desired, all of which enhance its effectiveness rate. FAM can be learnt from a teacher or via websites such as www.lizzieruffle.co.uk (Ruffell, 2011); www.fertilityuk.org (Fertility UK, 2002); www.fwhc.org (Feminist Women's Health Center, 2011).

These two natural methods get bad press, with jokes about their inefficiency or that women's cycles (women's bodies) are somehow too chaotic and unpredictable. Once taught to understand the basic infertile pattern and how to monitor and interpret the signs of the fertile stage (which takes only about three menstrual/fertility cycles), it is relatively easy to know when you are fertile and when you are not. Being aware of your fertility requires a higher degree of mindfulness about how you want to manage your fertility in relationship with your sexual behaviour: do you want to get pregnant, or avoid pregnancy either by not having unprotected intercourse, or by using a barrier method? Some believe that due to the consciousness involved in choosing these methods, users are far more conscientious about using them properly. Many statistics given for efficacy of contraceptives are based on laboratory trials about their "perfect" use as opposed to their, more often, "actual" use. A study at the University of California (UC Davis, 2011) shows, for example, that contraceptive pills typically have an eight per cent failure rate rather than the zero-point-three (0.3) per cent claimed. A longitudinal study on the efficacy of FAM was published in *Human Reproduction* (Frank-Herrmann et al., 2007). It was conducted in Germany and involved 900 women. The actual use of FAM (knowing your fertile phase and either avoiding genital contact, or using barrier methods during that time) resulted in 1.8% unintended pregnancies. Standard adjustments used to discover the "perfect" use rates suggested a 0.6% failure rate when there was no unprotected intercourse in the fertile phase.

Clearly, women (and men) have benefited by being free to have intercourse at any time without the risk of pregnancy, due to contraception. Rather than utilising our knowledge that women are fertile for only a short time in each cycle, we have developed a range of contraception to interrupt the natural hormonal cycle, many with side effects. Bennett and Pope (2008) explore many of the physical health and psychological issues surrounding the pill, including a range of wider social issues. They raise the question: how do we regard and respect our fertility? Shapiro (1987) argues that women get to feel that their fertility is a liability, in the way of sexual availability. She says the best contraceptives are seen as those that do not "interfere" with lovemaking, perhaps part of our romantic view of sex that it should be "spontaneous". It also promotes the idea that sex should include intercourse and intromission. One consequence is to put aside conscious choosing of sexual behaviours that could lead to pregnancy. Another is to undermine our awareness of practising safer sex to reduce the chances of sexually transmitted infections.

Exercise   Your fertility

Think about your experiences of your fertility.

As a woman, have you been pregnant when you didn't plan to be? How did you feel, what did you do, how do you feel now? Are you wanting to conceive and finding that difficult or undergoing fertility treatment? What is your experience of this? Have you lost a pregnancy or had a stillbirth?

As a man, how do you feel about your fertility? What experiences have you had of a woman being pregnant with your child or with any of the issues mentioned above?

Write about your experiences, how you feel about them now, and what impact this has on how you currently view your fertility. Consider how your views and experiences of fertility affect your feelings about your sexuality and your sexual behaviour.

The pleasure principle

If we think about how many thousands of babies are being born daily, we can get an idea of how many millions of sexual acts humans are engaging in. What are the motivations for, or needs of, all these other non-reproductive sexual acts? As a brief enquiry, I asked fifty people (colleagues and students who had attended various training days), "What do you like about sex?" There were four categories of reply.

1. *Pleasure*: For fun, excitement, affection, and the physical sensations of kissing, hugging, and orgasm; for relaxation or to relieve or release tension.
2. *Intimacy*: To share a bond with a partner; a love or spiritual connection; mutual healing.
3. *Emotional pleasure*: Joy and laughter, anticipation and exploration.
4. *Power*: For money or power-over; for empowerment (Figure 3).

Cormier-Otaño (2011a) outlines what he calls the five Ps of sex; that people have sex for any or a combination of the following reasons:

• pleasure (feel-good factor, inner chemistry);
• play (fun, expression, escapism, and creativity);
• procreation (existential needs);
• parallelism: a parallel experience of matching with another, being in unison;
• palliating effect (to relieve or lessen pain, alleviate stress, to re-balance).

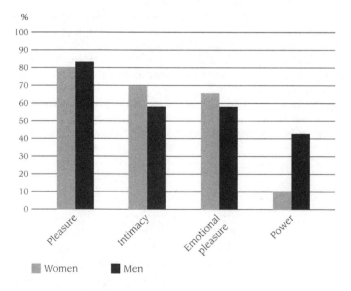

Figure 3. What do you like about sex?

What we are taught about pleasure, sexual intimacy, and our sexuality, as distinct from reproductive abilities, is limited. Our goal orientated view of sex implies a progression through activities, some desirable, some only to pave the way to allow for penetration/intercourse and thrusting, which should lead to (male) ejaculation/orgasm. This marginalises other sexual orientations and minimises the many other satisfying sexual behaviours people engage in as just "foreplay", or something somehow lesser than the real thing. It encourages the belief about sex as something we do, rather than about being a sexual person. A circular view of sex allows us to flow in and out of whichever behaviours we are in the mood for in whichever order we choose, bringing in, and allowing for, creativity and spontaneity in our sexual encounters (Figure 4).

Having "a sexuality", being a sexual being, includes a desire for pleasure and often a desire for other. It hooks our curiosity and our desires to play and have fun. Sexual desire is a reflex, a sexual energy charge in the body, causing many physiological changes and feelings and emotions. By becoming more conscious of our desire, what turns us on and what turns us off physically, emotionally, and psychologically, we become more aware of our feelings about these desires. When we are also more conscious about our values and beliefs about sexuality, we can consider options and make choices about which

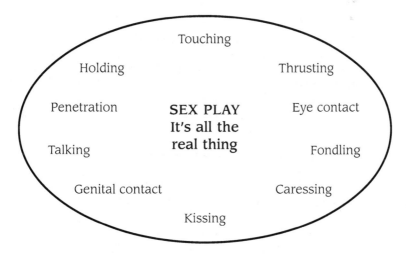

Figure 4.   A circular view of sexual play.

ways of expressing ourselves and which sexual behaviours will enhance our sexual self-esteem. Connecting more with the idea of being sexual, of sexuality as a subjective experience, we can see how objectifying our current perceptions are.

Exercise   Best and worst experiences

Note down your three best consensual sexual experiences

1.
2.
3.

Note down your three worst consensual sexual experiences

1.
2.
3.

Notice the memories: what images are triggered, what body sensations and what feelings. When you have noticed your reactive responses, take your attention to what you are thinking. Take some time to think about the differences. Is it about where you were, whom you were with, what you did, and what happened to you? Is there anything that you realise now that you didn't then?

Write down three things about your best sexual experience that made it so good

1.
2.
3.

Please note: this exercise may trigger memories, thoughts, and feelings about non-consensual experiences. If so, take some time to address this by going back to the exercise "Applying the brakes" (pp. xxxii–xxxiii). Take time to think and choose if and when you want to do this exercise.

Sex and power

There are many issues about sex and power that are addressed throughout this book. That sexuality is a powerful subject in itself is evidence of our need to discuss this sometimes uncomfortable issue. There are fine lines between pain and pleasure, and sex and sexuality are issues where we explore these arenas deeply, both physically and emotionally.

Many are reviewing our individual and social relationships to power. The old models of power are about power-over, about dominance, about someone winning and someone losing. Macy and Young Brown (1998) say that within a power-over model, we believe rigidity and armouring make us more powerful, whereas they actually restrict our vision and movement. They say this model is dysfunctional to the social system because it inhibits diversity and feedback mechanisms, and, thus, fosters systemic disintegration. Open systems, however, maintain a balance amid constant change and evolve in complexity by adapting to their environment. Within the homeodynamic model, feedback loops are integral to self-regulation, to our self-organising processes.

The "drama triangle", developed and reworked by Karpman (1968), outlines three positions which people have learnt to use as ways to relate to others: the Persecutor, the Rescuer and the Victim. They are interdependent and often leave one with a sense of frustration. These roles are usually unconscious behaviour patterns, often developed in childhood, and very common in our society. We use a phrase, *drama queen*, for people who regularly seem to have some chaos going on in their lives. People who grow up in highly adrenalised environments as children, with parents who fight frequently, or who are addicts, or mentally unstable, for example, will often be predisposed in this way. The section titled "Brain" will discuss this subject in more depth. Recognising whether we play these roles can alert us to dynamics in our relationships and allow us to reconsider how we could behave more honestly, yet with compassion for others.

- The Persecutor is a bully who has anger as the main emotion, a frustrator who attempts to achieve inner peace by going to war. These people are blaming, critical, and often enjoy conflict. They need Victims or Rescuers to hide their own fears and vulnerabilities, and project hostility on to others to justify their defensiveness. They might be aggressive in their choice of language and tone and pitch of voice. In contrast, when being assertive, we might well stand our ground and speak up for ourselves, but in a manner that can be heard and received by another.
- The Rescuer is a people-pleaser, someone who wants to help. They frustrate by creating a world of good but helpless people; they need Victims and can easily switch into a bullying role. They

have guilt as a dominant emotion, have difficulty saying no and maintaining boundaries, and often feel taken for granted. Rather than helping *per se*, their motivation is to get self-esteem from being seen as warm, kind, and caring. If we do things that we do not really want to do, we can end up feeling resentful. Having true concern for others includes not taking over or doing more than your share, but only what is actually asked of you.

- The Victim is passive and wants to be told what to do; they complain but do not take action. They leave us feeling helpless and impotent as they ask for advice, but then say "Yes, but . . .". They often think the world owes them a living and can switch to bullying if not rescued. They have shame and pity as dominant emotions. There are obviously people who are vulnerable and have been victimised, which they recognise and are able to ask clearly for help and support.

Authors such as Elworthy (1991) and Starhawk (1990) have offered alternative approaches to power that are now the basis of mediation and conflict resolution programmes. Other perceptions of power could be having confidence in oneself and one's abilities, or having a good sense of self-esteem. The importance of people taking their power, but not abusing it, is crucial, from the therapist holding the boundaries of the therapeutic space, to the parents providing a secure base for the child, to the political leaders doing what they were elected to do. When the boundaries are held, with responsibility and respect, a win–win scenario can be created.

Assertive communication requires us to acknowledge our own and others' vulnerabilities, and to have compassion and empathy for others, but also for ourselves. An assertive person is aware of, and can separate, their own thoughts, feelings, and motivations, and can distinguish between "can't" and "don't want to". They can manage conflict and weigh up contradictions; they can think and reflect before taking action. They can stay with their own opinion without needing to criticise or become defensive. Being assertive includes being willing to negotiate and share skills and resources. This is discussed further in the section titled "Relationships".

People who have experienced abuse of power can find it difficult to step into their own authority, fearing that they, too, might abuse their power. Others replay power abuse, which, from a psychotherapeutic perspective, could be an unconscious compulsion to repeat or to normalise previous experiences. There is much to be gained through sexual empowerment and much to be lost through sexual violation. In order to discuss sexual self-esteem in the widest sense, we need to think about our relationships to power: to our own power, to the power of our sexuality, and to consider wielding the sword of power with care.

Exercise   Sexual timeline

Think about your sexual experiences from your first consensual experience up until now. Draw a timeline and identify up to ten experiences. Don't go into details, but briefly note what has brought each one to mind. Was it the place, the person, and/or what happened that has made it memorable?

When you have written your timeline, look at it overall; can you see any patterns? Did most events happen at a particular age? Was it with a specific person or types of people? Was it what happened mostly that has made these events significant? Notice which of these things is most important to you (where, who, or how).

Consider what you have written in this exercise with regard to issues of power as discussed above. Does the "'Drama triangle" feel familiar to you? If so, how? How have issues of power been a part of your (consensual) sexual history? Is there anything you want to change in the future, and if so, how would you want to do that?

Looking good

There is obviously great pleasure to be found in expressing our sexuality through attending to our appearance with clothes, make-up, and accessories and having fun playing with all this. Many derive great pleasure from playing with materials, different fabrics, colours, and shapes. Many enjoy designing outfits, trying different styles and fashions. Much fun is had by groups of women, in the hours spent together "getting ready" to go out, swapping ideas, clothes, and accessories. Culturally, we are bombarded with media and images about looking good and what looks good. We are encouraged to think more about what we look like to others and how we might appeal to them rather than to what makes us feel sensual and sexual. We are encouraged to use (and abuse) our sexual power; our power to attract, to get what we want.

Despite the average British woman being a size fourteen, a recent television programme (*Miss Naked Beauty*, 2008) showed that most mannequins in High Street shops are a size ten. Most women and many men have a low opinion of their body image and many are caught in cycles of dieting and eating disorders. Our current sexualised image for women is quite distorted. It is almost as if what is admired as beauty in women is a very thin girl, with no body hair but very large bust, like our Barbie dolls, whose proportions are actually ridiculous. In ratio to the average woman's waist size, her bra size is thirty-eight EE and she is eight feet ten inches tall! There is much pressure on men these days, too, about body image and sexual prowess. Writers such as Zilbergeld (1992), have challenged ideas that men are supposed to be "hard as steel and go all night", and Biddulph (2004) also has discussed the pressures of rigid sex role stereotypes and their impact on male physical and emotional health.

There is a great deal of focus on our imperfections and hundreds of products to buy to improve our sexual attractiveness. We are encouraged to feel ashamed, not proud, of the bodies we have, which do, after all, come in many different shapes and sizes. The lengths to which we are encouraged to go for the sake of beauty have become increasingly severe, such as extreme dieting and cosmetic procedures. Obviously, being physically healthy improves our feel-good factor, but being attractive is more to do with feeling attractive, feeling physically and emotionally good about yourself.

Ironically, there are also serious questions about the potential health risks of many "health and beauty" products because of some of the ingredients. The Women's Environmental Network (2006) has carried out research to indicate the most worrying examples, and also to highlight how commonly they are used. There are 30,000–100,000 chemicals used in cosmetics, with ninety-five per cent of them having little or no health or environmental safety information. The word "Parfum" is used to describe between fifty and one hundred different chemical fragrances.

The two most widely used compounds are parabens and phthalates (DiGangi & Norin, 2002). Parabens are used in many cosmetics and products, such as shampoos, bubble-bath, shower gels, make-up, lotions, and deodorants. (Have a look at the ingredients of items that you have.) They have been detected in human breast tissue and, although they cannot yet be conclusively linked as a possible cause of breast cancer, evidence now suggests they can act as oestrogen mimics. There is concern about the huge rise in breast cancer rates; the numbers have doubled in twenty years, with the causes of 50–70% of cases classed as "unknown". One paraben (propyl paraben) has been shown to adversely affect male reproductive functions. At the "daily intake level" currently acceptable under EC law, it decreased daily sperm production.

Phthalates are linked to reproductive damage, and some have been banned because of this. They are commonly found in products such as deodorants, fragrances, hair gels, hair sprays and mousses, and hand and body lotions. Many couples now suffer with fertility problems and many women have diseases associated with hormone disruption, such as irregular menstrual cycles, polycystic ovaries, endometriosis, and fibroids. There has also been a huge rise in prostate cancer incidence over the last twenty years. Cancer Research UK (2008) says it is now the most common cancer in men in Britain, accounting for nearly a quarter of all new male cancer diagnoses. There is concern that these issues are correlated not just to lifestyle factors, but also to toxicity in foods and our environment.

There are two reports by the Women's Environmental Network, "Getting lippy" and "Pretty nasty" (Budd et al., 2003) which provide more details, including how to avoid these compounds and some alternative health and beauty products. Some of their suggestions are:

- never mix cosmetics—such as remnants of your old shampoo with the contents of a new bottle—as they may not be made to be mixed with other chemicals; this may lead to formation of nitrosamines;
- never allow cosmetics to exceed their "best before" date—if there is not one listed it means the product has been formulated to have a minimum shelf-life of thirty months;
- wear less make-up! Try having a day without make-up and note people's reactions;
- use your consumer choice to buy products which are simply formulated and as ecologically sound as possible. Every time you choose a cleaner product you send a vote to the makers;
- use some of the easy, natural alternatives, instead of the manufactured products;
- try to avoid synthetic fragrances and perfumes, and opt for diluted essential oils instead;

- call for the substitution of potentially harmful chemical ingredients with GM-free herbal or plant-based alternatives with a proven safety record, and support the development of alternative testing methods;
- beware of the pressures of glossy advertising and exploitative media images.

Exercise   Beautiful body

Use your "Safe space", as described above (pp. xxxii–xxxiii). Make it warm.

Sit for a few moments and close your eyes. Allow your breath to settle. Allow sounds and distractions to just come and go. Think about your body, your breathing lungs, your beating heart, your brain and bones, muscles, torso, and limbs. Feel any sensations in your body, consciously tense and then relax.

Put your left hand on your heart area and your right hand on your stomach and give yourself a chance to relax your body and breathing . . . Imagine you have just woken up in your body. For the first time you realise you are inside this body. You are excited and curious. You are told you are the first woman, the first man ever. You are the prototype that all future humans will be modelled on.

Get up, take your clothes off, look at yourself naked in a full-length mirror. What do you see? Look front and back and from the side, take your time. Look at yourself from all angles as if you haven't seen a human body before. Move yourself, your limbs. Be aware of what you, this body, is and what it can do.

Notice if there are any aspects of your body you don't like and any that you do like.

Be aware of your feelings and thoughts about yourself. Notice if you are kind, appreciative, and accepting of your body, or whether you are critical.

If you are critical, perhaps you could plan how you could make some changes to what you don't like through exercise or dietary alterations, for example. If you can't or don't want to do that, consider how you could you love yourself just as you are.

Sexual identity

We commonly use the phrase sexual identity to mean a person's sexual orientation. Because we implicitly use a reproductive model of sex, it implies a heterosexual model; therefore, people who are not heterosexual by orientation or identification have been defined and labelled as "other". Scientists have tried to discover why people are sexually attractive to, and attracted by, some people and not others, and why some are attracted to the same sex and some not. They have tested many theories exploring whether sexual attraction might be based on facial shapes, hormones, pheromones, psychological profiling, or on reproductive qualities. None seems to be proved, except that a spark of attraction happens within seconds of people meeting. It seems that the reflex in the brain just happens; who we see, fancy, or respond to, is a reaction. This spark of attraction sets off a whole neurochemical, hormonal, physiological reaction in our bodies.

There are many labels such as straight, lesbian, gay, bisexual, transgender/sexual, kink, queer, polyamorous, and so on. They serve to identify sexual orientations and lifestyles other than heterosexual, but they are not homogenous groups and vary in interpretation and expression. For some, identifying with a group or with a particular sexual identity is very important: it is about belonging, a political statement, or a vital part of their self-identity. There are many people who accept the notion of sexual diversity and sexual fluidity. In the 2011 annual Integrated Household Survey (Sherwin, 2011), a question giving a choice of sexual identities showed the largest increase in the "Don't know" answers, rather than people choosing one answer. But others do not accept diversity and pathologise any sexual identities that are not heterosexual. This leads to a power differential with social and legal implications. Non-heterosexuals have to "come out" to family, friends, and colleagues, not knowing whether they will be accepted or rejected, whether they might be at risk of losing relationships or jobs. Others are at risk of bullying or violence.

Kort (2003) says "coming out" involves a process including recognising, accepting, expressing, and sharing one's sexual orientation with oneself and others. He has adapted the model of gay and lesbian identity formation, developed by Vivienne Cass in 1979, to identify several phases that people might go through:

1. *Identity confusion*: personalisation of information regarding sexuality.
   - Recognises thought/behaviours as homosexual, usually finds this unacceptable.
   - Redefines meaning of behaviours.
   - Seeks information on homosexuality.
2. *Identity comparison*: accepts possibility s/he might be homosexual.
   - Feels positive about being different, exhibits this in ways beyond orientation.

- Accepts behaviour as homosexual, rejects homosexual identity.
- Accepts identity but inhibits behaviour (e.g., heterosexual marriage/anonymous sex).

3. *Identity tolerance*: accepts probability of being homosexual, recognises sexual/social/emotional needs of being homosexual.
   - Seeks out meeting other gay/lesbian people through groups, bars, etc.
   - Personal experience builds sense of community, positively and negatively.

4. *Identity acceptance*: accepts (*vs.* tolerates) homosexual self-image and has increased contact with gay/lesbian subculture and less with heterosexuals.
   - Increased anger towards anti-gay society.
   - Greater self-acceptance.

5. *Identity pride*: immersed in gay/lesbian subculture, less interaction with heterosexuals. Views world divided as "gay" or "not gay".
   - Confrontation with heterosexual establishment.
   - Disclosure to family, co-workers.

6. *Identity synthesis*: gay/lesbian identity integrated with other aspects.
   - Recognises supportive heterosexual others.
   - Sexual identity still important, but not primary factor in relationships with others.

Kaufman and Raphael (1996) believe that sexual orientation is affected by three factors: first, a person's erotic attraction—who is it who catches your eye? Second, who do you yearn to touch and hold, in that affection communicates protection and security, which is the foundation for trust? And third, identification: who you wish to be intimate with, share fusion and merging; whose eyes do you want to gaze into? Diamond (2008) has shown, through her study of women, that for many, love and desire are not rigidly heterosexual or homosexual, but fluid and changeable, through various stages of life and social groups and, most importantly, different love relationships. Cormier-Otaño (2011b) has conducted some interesting research around asexuality, where individuals want many of the aspects of being "in relationships" but do not want to be sexual. They might want to be intimate and affectionate, but, rather than "suffering" from low sexual desire, many are choosing a sexual identity of being asexual. This challenges our social assumptions around sexual desire: that everyone wants to be sexual, or, at least, should want to. Asexuality challenges our assumptions that low sexual desire is in itself a dysfunction.

Swami and Furnham (2008) have explored a wider idea of what they call "dynamic attractiveness", where they found people are actually more interested in a person's conversational and social skills, personality, and sense of humour. How we think and feel about our reflexive reactions will also influence our response to our attractions. Sometimes we act on our sexual feelings, and sometimes not. Some people choose celibacy and/or chastity as a lifestyle and some feel socially or culturally uncomfortable with their sexual orientation, so do not express this aspect of themselves at all. Moving away from a hetero-normative view would reduce the need for labelling, resulting in a situation where sexual identity could be more widely understood as describing our desire, sexual tastes, and preferences. It could include what we believe and identify with to suit our sensuality and feelings and our sexual values. Our sexual identity is also about our experience of our passions and creativity, as well as our choices of behaviour and lifestyle.

Exercise   Sexual preferences

Write down five things that you are easily aware of that you prefer sexually. They might be who you are attracted to or sexual behaviours you like.

1.
2.
3.
4.
5.

Write down five more things that you have discovered are part of what you prefer sexually from the earlier exercise about your best sexual experiences.

1.
2.
3.
4.
5.

Food for thought

Food is a good analogy when talking about sexuality, as both involve our mouths and lips, and both are about our tastes; what we like and what we do not like. Sexual arousal stimulates a desire to use our mouths, to kiss and taste, as well as touch. Hunger and the sexual drive are both urges/needs, linked to the pleasure centres in the brain, and trigger the release of dopamine and oxytocin, feel-good hormones. Both of these subjects are also culturally complex and deeply emotive, bringing a range of conditions and health issues. Food means so much more to us than satisfying our need to stay alive; we can derive great pleasure in choosing and preparing food, as well as eating it. We also often share food and eating as a social and bonding experience.

There is a huge range of different foods available for us to eat and, also, lots of different sexual behaviours. Different people like different foods, and we have differing sexual tastes. We have different cultural preferences in the same ways that some foods are seasonal and some only grow in certain countries because of different climates. Some foods are nutritious and great for health and some not, some give us a quick sugar rush that later depletes the body. Is this also true for sexual behaviours, and if so, which ones and why? What sort of ingredients would be part of a healthy sexual diet and what sort of sexual diet do we want?

To think about the analogy of food and how we express our sexuality, we need to consider the physiology: why we need food/sex, and how the body metabolises or might use sexual "nutrients"? Which might be toxic and why, and how might they affect us? In the "Body" section, we will consider the impacts of sexuality on our whole body, and in the "Brain" section, the hormones and neurochemicals involved. In the section titled "Emotion", we will discuss the interplay

---

Exercise   How do you nourish yourself?

Think about your favourite meal and what it is you like about it. For example, it could be the foods, how they are prepared, or in what combinations. How nourishing is your meal as a food source?

Now imagine this meal was a sexual encounter: what can this tell you about what you like and what you want sexually? Is there any correlation between how you nourish yourself with food and how you feed yourself sexually?

of all of these factors and how we might begin to answer the question of what is a healthy sexual diet.

We need also to think about the preparation of food: which ingredients to use and how we want to use or prepare them, what cooking or seasoning we might want to use. The presentation of food and the ambience in which we eat, or express ourselves sexually, will influence our experiences as well. And, as always, someone has to clean up afterwards. Rather than promoting any particular "diet", this book encourages the reader to explore the issues and then decide which tastes and choices suit them.

Sexual values

"Sexual values" seems to be an old-fashioned phrase, but what if we were to reclaim the concept to ask, what do we actually value? What is valuable to us in terms of our belief systems, our bodies, minds, and hearts? We can consider the huge range of behaviours and human expressions of sexuality that we know about and draw up a set of our own values to live by. We can decide individually what we value for ourselves, what we think is all right for others, but not to our taste. We can also think more socially and culturally about what we do not think is valuable for ourselves or for others.

As a society, we would see more clearly how sexual prejudice has been enshrined in our laws, including the criminalisation of some gay adult consensual behaviour. Becoming more explicit about our cultural beliefs and assumptions would also help to challenge our contradictory attitudes to crimes of sexual violence. On the one hand, rape is considered a serious crime with a long-term sentence; on the other hand, in practice, many victims choose not to report it, knowing they will go through an arduous process where conviction rates are as low as six per cent (Holden, 2008).

We have a cultural ambivalence towards sexual violence, where we glorify it through pornography and normalise it as entertainment in mainstream cinema and television shows. We still often blame victims by enquiring about what they might have done to deserve it; were they dressed or behaving in a sexual manner, drunk, or out late alone (Amnesty International, 2005)? The natural ability to go through a recovery process after a traumatic event can be compromised by this attitude, where victims continue to blame themselves, too. This can contribute to the development of sexual problems and post traumatic stress disorder.

By being clearer about our choices and preferences, we can evaluate the range of sexual behaviours and lifestyle choices, and decide for ourselves what is important for us when we consider these issues all together. We can evaluate our sexual appetite and decide on our own sexual diet. We can become more proud of who we are, creatively express our sexuality, and develop a good sense of sexual self-esteem.

Exercise   Sexual values

Write down five ways you have expressed your sexuality in the past week, whatever they may be.

1.
2.
3.
4.
5.

Then read the list below of some of the different ways in which people express their sexuality through sexual acts and behaviours and lifestyles. Add some more if you wish.

Expressions of sexuality

Anal sex	Bondage and dominance
Buying sex	Celibacy
Chat lines	Child pornography
Clitoral stimulation	Cuddling
Dogging	Dressing up
Dry penetration	Erotic dancing
Fisting	Faithful to one person
Fucking	Initiating sexual encounters
Kink	Kissing
Massage	Masturbation
Oral sex	Rimming
Sado-masochism	Selling sex
Sex as a spiritual experience	Sex in groups
Sex for procreation	Sex in private
Sex in public places	Sex only if married
Sex parties	Sex only with people you love
Sex shops	Sex toys
Sex with animals	Sex with multiple partners

Sex with opposite sex	Sex with same sex
Sex with strangers	Sex for procreation
Sharing sexual fantasies	Snogging
Stroking	Swinging
Talking during sex	Vaginal intercourse
Viewing illegal pornography	Viewing legal pornography

Now take some time to really think about the words sexual *values*, as in what is valuable to you, of importance or useful.

Make a page with three columns with the headings:

What I value for myself	What I don't value for myself but *do* value for others	What I don't value for myself and *do not* value for others

Write each of the above sexual expressions in one of the three columns, according to what you think and feel about them. You may want to go by your first reaction or consider each and choose where you want to place them.

Have a look at your lists; what is it like to see these distinctions? How do you feel about what you really do value for yourself? How do you feel about those that you don't think have value?

Of the things that you don't value for yourself, but can see are valuable for others, consider whether this is about your beliefs or preferences, or whether they are behaviours you might like to experiment with in the future.

Your values might change over time; you may want to do this exercise again at the end of the book. You might identify values you have which no longer suit you and wish to set about changing them.

Sex, love, and relationships

We have reviewed some of our beliefs and thinking about sex, including our procreative needs and the pleasures of human sexuality. Let us now consider emotional and intimacy issues. If our sexual desire is often triggered by an "other", creating a want to reach out, to kiss or touch them, what are our relational needs from sex and our sexuality? These are important issues to consider given our attitudes that sex is something we do; that we make love *to* someone, rather than *with* them. Relational issues also question our cultural objectification of sexuality, that we should look attractive *to* someone rather than *feel* sexual, and our increasing normalisation of depersonalised sex.

Much has been written about sex and intimacy, specifically about our early attachment relationships and their effects on our future choices of partners and our abilities to sustain sexual relationships as adults. Putting together the model of stages of development by

Hendrix (1995) with Kaufman and Raphael's (1996) outline of basic interpersonal needs (shown in italics) allows us to consider the development of sexual self-esteem.

Need for touching and holding
Attachment, leading to emotional security

Our need for relationships with other people is significant in the first stage, which Hendrix calls "attachment". We reach out for touching and holding. As infants, we need someone to feed us and nurture us or we will die. We reach first with our mouths for food, then, as we can grasp, we move whatever we touch to our mouths, where we taste and, given our nose is so near, probably smell, too. Attachment is the beginning of our social bonding, where the sense of sight is also vital, the importance of seeing and being seen.

When the infant's gaze is met with a smile (the facial expression of joy) from the primary care-giver, it is soothed and will experience emotional security. If it is met with anger or indifference, it will feel distress and react through one of the survival circuits of fight, flight, or panic. Essentially, each interaction will induce either our reward system or our survival circuits. The feelings of pleasure will activate the reward system and release feel-good neurochemicals such as serotonin or oxytocin. Alternatively, our distress will induce feelings of pain and activate our survival system, prompting the release of adrenalin and cortisol. Gerhardt (2004) describes in detail how brain development is affected by our early experiences and why, indeed, love matters so much. She also explains the harm that can be done physically to our neurochemical patterning and our nervous system, and psychologically to our emotional well-being, and, therefore, socially, affecting our expectations and capacities in adult relationships.

If, in the first year and a half of our life, our attachment needs are adequately met, we will have a biochemical pattern of feeling pleasure, and, therefore, expect to receive pleasure when we reach out to someone to be in relationship with them, to be touched and held. We will have achieved an internal sense of emotional security, leading to a fundamental belief in our right to exist, in our desires to reach out, and a trust in other people that they will respond positively. During the attachment phase, the infant decides through its experiences with parents and carers whether relationships are trustworthy or not (Erikson, 1959). If our needs are not met, our biochemical pattern is one of stress hormones and the need for survival reactions, leading to emotional insecurity. Maybe here we learn a sense of shame about our need for others.

Within the arena of sexuality, our wants and needs for attachment, for touching and holding, are not valued in our society. The fact that we desire another, who we want to kiss and feel, is rarely acknow-ledged. We do not seem to teach or encourage these needs as primary; rather, we focus on sexual acts and sexual positions. Hite (1994) noted that when researching what people liked about being sexual, there was one activity that many people mentioned that we have no quick phrase or word to describe: lying alongside their lover, naked, kissing, holding each other, and feeling their whole bodies touching, while they looked into each other's eyes.

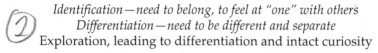

Identification—need to belong, to feel at "one" with others
Differentiation—need to be different and separate
Exploration, leading to differentiation and intact curiosity

The second phase is exploration, between eighteen months and three years old. The child can now move independently and explore the world around them. Encouragement to discover their world (along with guidelines about obvious dangers) will promote an intact curiosity and a sense of differentiation. During the exploration phase, the child is developing autonomy and self-worth or a sense of shame, of low self-esteem which can lead to self-doubt and a feeling of not being able to rely on anything or anyone.

Another way we are often shamed sexually is through adults' responses to children touching their genitals. There is a natural incli-nation for children to do this; it is a form of self-soothing. Parents often discourage their children from doing this, especially in public, telling them it is bad or dirty. Depending on the degree of shaming that continues as the child grows, this can lead to shame about masturbation and other forms of self-pleasuring as an adult.

This exploration phase is activated during sexual attraction when we become curious about someone and want to get to know them or more about them. Feeling shame about our curiosity, having been dis-couraged about "wanting to know", or ridiculed for asking questions, will dampen our sense of inquisitiveness. It might discourage us as adults from acting on our attractions or desires.

We also have a need at this stage for identification, to belong and feel at "one" with others, but also to be different and separate. How much we have been encouraged and allowed to do this as children will influence our capacity to accept ourselves and also our tolerance about the differences that others have from us.

Need for power in our relationships and in our lives
Identity, leading to secure sense of self

The third phase is identity. Aged between three and four years, the child begins to assert these differences. If they are accepted and still kept in attachment, that is, not rejected for these differences, they will feel supported to have a unique sense of identity, and develop a secure sense of self. For example, are they allowed to show personal preferences for food or clothing? We have a need for power in our relationships and in our lives. This does not mean power over others, but a sense of personal power, such as the right to choose, to want something different, or feel something different from others.

This is important for a sense of sexual self-esteem, particularly for people of minority sexual identities and sexual preferences, as their ability to fend off homophobia, internally and externally, might be strengthened or weakened by how strongly their sense of self has been allowed to develop around this age. This phase can also have an impact on our ability to feel individuated in relationship, which can lead to power struggles and conflict in friendships and work relationships, as well as with sexual partners.

Affirmation—need to feel worthwhile, valued and admired
Competence, leading to sense of personal power to achieve

The fourth phase is competence, where the four- to seven-year-old focuses on competing. If affirmed, valued, admired, and made to feel worthwhile, the child will experience a sense of personal power in its right and ability to succeed and achieve. We are learning to master our world; reading and writing, developing physical skills such as sports or playing an instrument, or learning to be in relationships, learning to share and to negotiate and accommodate between what we want and what others want or need. The more we receive support and empathy from others—our carers, parents, and peers—about our struggles and difficulties in developing these skills, the more sympathetic and less critical we will be of ourselves and of others.

This stage is intrinsic to a sense of self-worth, of being seen and valued for the unique human being that you are. Difficulties in this phase can undermine a growing sense of being all right, of valuing your own uniqueness, your own body shape and attributes. Current cultural body shaming and desires for cosmetic surgery would indicate that many were not allowed to develop successfully through this stage.

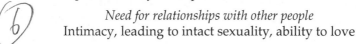

Need to nurture, care for, and help others
Concern, leading to concern for others

Between seven and thirteen years old, we learn to sympathise, to feel concern for others. We have a need to nurture, to care for and help others. Our abilities to empathise are vital for successful social and sexual relationships. Seven is also seen as the age at which we begin to develop a consciousness, an awareness about what is happening around us. We become more aware of what people say and do and how this makes us, and others, feel.

The ability to empathise, to be able to step into another's world and imagine what it is like from their perspective, is vital for good relationships. The ability to empathise with ourselves and our human imperfections is vital, too. Difficulties through this stage can lead to the development of a strong critical stance towards the self, and, therefore, usually also towards others. This can lead to perfectionist traits, which, due to the impossibility of achieving perfection, can leave someone with a sense of failure or of never being good enough, and nothing and no one ever good enough for them. Again, this is evident in our culture, with our media encouraging us to always look for more, for bigger, for better. A lack of feeling that ourselves, our relationships, or our things are "good enough" can lead to a general sense of discontentment, of lack of satiation, and, ultimately, an addiction or compulsion to try to be perfect.

Need for relationships with other people
Intimacy, leading to intact sexuality, ability to love

In the final phase in Hendrix's model, between thirteen and nineteen years old, we are developing our needs for intimacy and our developmental behaviour is integrating. Successful transition through this stage will lead to an intact sexuality and an ability to love. At this stage of sexual development, how our carers, parents, and peers respond will be vital in developing a sense of sexual self-esteem.

This must be confusing to young people, given our cultural ambivalence to sexuality. On the one hand, they live in an environment with a highly sexualised media, with sex being used to sell just about everything. On the other hand, there is little celebration about sexuality; what an amazing gift we have to be able to experience sexual pleasure in our bodies or through sharing sexually with another. If adults do not feel comfortable about their own sexuality, they will find it difficult to openly discuss and support or promote and celebrate their children's emerging sexuality. Many young people are turning to pornography to fill the gaps in their education about adult sexuality and sexual relationships, which does not focus on intimacy, on negotiating and integrating the needs of the self and another.

This stage brings together all the other developmental phases. Successful transitions through the phases will motivate the reward system, the feel-good neurochemicals such as dopamine and serotonin. We will feel accepting of our basic needs and confident that generally they will be received and accepted by others. Difficulties through these stages can lead to a preponderance of stress hormones as the survival brain circuits are more often activated. This, in turn, can lead to a reduction in our frontal lobe development, affecting our ability to think things through, evaluate, and make choices. We might feel intrinsically ashamed about our basic needs, and, being human, have developed coping strategies to get our needs met. As adults, these strategies can, and do, become outmoded and can undermine our ability to have successful social relationships. Difficulties in social relating obviously affect our abilities to have sustaining and fulfilling sexual relationships.

A main principle of this book is relationships, the internal interplay between our reactive brain and/or reflective mind, and the dialogue between these and our body and our feelings. This section has explored some of our social and cultural issues in our relationship to human sexuality, and how, as individuals, we relate to ourselves and others, including family, community, friends, and lovers. Another facet that humans like about sexuality is sexual love and having sexual relationships. They might start from a sexual attraction that leads to a sexual encounter that develops into a sexual relationship, which might then lead on to marriage, civil partnership, or living together, being flatmates, companions, friends, and maybe co-parenting. Or they might start from a friendship or work relationship that develops into a sexual relationship. Love is a subject that fascinates us and is a wonderful part of being human. What exactly love is has been a question of debate for centuries. Love takes many forms that are non-sexual, such as loving our family, children, friends, or animals. It makes us feel good and can bring great joy and delight. When things go wrong in our love relationships, it can also bring deep distress and heartache.

Some people want and deeply enjoy the intimacy that develops through having sex with the same person again and again and others prefer sexual encounters with different people. At different stages or times in our lives we might want either, or both! We might have dilemmas about wanting to experience the intimacy of one emotionally deep sexual partnership while also desiring variety in our sexual encounters. Whatever we choose, we can still be in good relationship with ourselves; we can be embodied and conscious. Becoming clearer about our sexual beliefs and values, our tastes and our desires for sexual relationships, encourages us to be more selective, to choose the type of sexual encounters or relationships that we want and value, the types of sexual expression that will nurture our bodies, hearts, and souls.

Exercise   Sex, love, and relationships

Write down something/s that you *believe* about the following:

Sexual relationships

Sex and love

Love and relationships

Sex and love and relationships

What if . . .?

What if we were to begin to think differently about sexuality? What if we were to become more mindful, to re-evaluate and recreate our mind-set, our thinking and beliefs, and more consciously redefine what we think individually, culturally, and socially? For example, sex education could teach detailed sexual anatomy and physiology, as distinct from reproduction, including the stages and processes involved in sexual attraction and arousal. Knowing what our sexual processes are helps us to understand what might be happening if something goes wrong; knowing ourselves sexually would give us a clearer idea of what we might need to put things right again. What if we were taught about fertility awareness as teenagers, so that we could make more conscious choices about our fertility and also about our sexual behaviour with regard to our thoughts and feelings about reproduction? Sexual health could mean more than merely the prevention of pregnancy and sexual infections, but could include our feelings and emotional health. Safer sex issues could also address physical safety and emotional well-being, and include related subjects like drugs and alcohol. The notion of sexual identity could include our sexual orientations and preferences, along with our beliefs and feelings and our choices about lifestyle and sexual behaviours.

We can think about "what if" because another advantage to humans having frontal lobes in the brain is the ability to imagine, to contemplate, to make believe. Maybe we can imagine the future, because we can also remember the past. Humans learn through the memory centres in the back brain. We can think to ourselves, "If I do this, then that might happen". We can weigh up consequences; we can, and do, learn though making mistakes, realising we might want to do something different next time. We can create because we can conceptualise and imagine what has not been seen or done before. We have changed, affected, and manipulated our environment in a way no other species on this planet has done before, for better and for worse.

Sexual imagination, the ability to fantasise, is a crucial aspect of healthy sexual functioning, as it enhances the arousal process and fuels the mind–brain–body–emotion circuit. Curiosity, anticipation, the excitement of looking forward to something, can all be aspects of foreplay. Critical thinking, worry, or anxiety can break the circuit of sexual arousal. Thinking about or replaying a previous sexual experience in our minds, in our imagination, can, and often will, trigger the sexual arousal reflex. Many people think sexual fantasy means having wild imaginings that we should probably be ashamed of, but research shows that the most pleasurable sexual fantasies will usually include things that please our beliefs and emotions, as well as our bodies (Friday, 1994; Kahr, 2007). Exploring our favourite or most common fantasies can help to deepen our understanding of our deepest desires by finding also the non-erotic themes and potentials from the details (Kort, 2011; Morin, 1996). Sexual fantasy is private; we can imagine whatever we like. For some, imagination is a place to explore things we might not want actually to do, or to consider if we did, how and where, and with whom.

So, what if we were to imagine and to begin to think about a health model for sexuality, to address our sexual health in the way that we do now concerning our physical health? We now understand the need for, and the benefits of, a good diet, physical exercise, and positive thinking, and we are mostly aware of the deleterious effect of unhealthy food, constant worrying, and the impact of modern stress on our well-being. But what do we know or think about what a healthy sexual diet or sexual appetite actually is or should be? Nourishment comforts us and provides us with what we need to grow (Roth, 1993). We need to hear and respect our individual and social needs for sexual health and well-being.

What if we were to include a more respectful, maybe spiritual or philosophical, approach to our sexuality as well, where we honour our sexuality and cherish our physical bodies and our hearts? Such attitudes embrace love and affection, the subjective experience of rela-tionship, of relating to our own sensuality and sexuality and to that of others. The pleasure principle promotes empowerment, encouraging respect for our bodies and our emotional well-being. We are aware these days of ecology and environmentalism, with many being more conscious about what energy sources we have on this planet, what we do to utilise them, and what side effects there are. Many are more aware of the short-term and long-term consequences of what and how we consume, and the important of re-evaluating our behaviours. What if we were to consider the ecology of our sexual energy? We could value our sexuality as a precious power resource to be used wisely. Our thoughts, feelings, and sexual practices, rather than being polluting or harmful to us, could be harnessed to enhance our well-being and our sexual health.

It is intrinsic in this book to ask these questions and to offer ideas and self-reflective exercises to provide some answers. A very common question asked about sexuality is "Am I normal?" By exploring each section, the reader can evaluate this for themselves. There is a huge diversity in human sexuality and what is desirable and preferable is unique to each individual. This section, the Mind, offers an opportu-nity to evaluate your beliefs, values, and choices. The Body section explores sensuality and the physiology of sexuality, and the Brain section our reflective urges. The section titled "Emotion" considers the emotional impact of our sexual beliefs, behaviours, and sexual expressions, including the impact on our bodies of sexualised trauma. The new model of this book is to understand ourselves more individually within each of these dimensions: our physical, emotional, and spiritual needs and desires, and to see how each affect and are affected by the others. *LoveSex* aims to promote a more consciously integrated sense of sexual self-esteem for individuals and for us as a society.

Exercise   Review of Part I

Read back through the exercises for this section and what you have written in your journal. Take some time to reflect on your exploration and to evaluate your work. Which exercises did you like and which ones did you not like? Think about why.

What have you discovered about your beliefs about sexuality, your sexual knowledge and where you got it from?

What have you discovered about your relationship to your body and how you nourish and value yourself, your sexual preferences and sexual values?

Is there anything that has surprised you? If so, how come? What is different than you had previously thought, and how do you feel about that?

Is there anything you want to change? If so, how could you do that?

Are there any exercises that you would like to do again? If so, notice what is similar or different if you do them a second time.

Talk to someone, write or draw something about how you are thinking and feeling having worked on this section.

PART II

BODY: SEXUAL ANATOMY

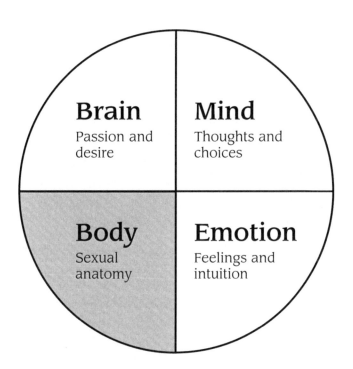

Body, brain, mind, and emotion.

The body

Inside out

In this section, we will explore our bodies and our sexual anatomy. Most of us know something about our reproductive functioning, at least a bit about periods, erections, ejaculation, and the mechanics of sexual intercourse. As children we are introduced to sex as something humans do to reproduce, which is, of course, true, but not the only reason we have sex. We are surprisingly ignorant about our sexual arousal process and our physical sexual functioning. We are not very well informed about the specifics of our fertility either. Here, we will clarify the differences between our reproductive and sexual processes and explore the different body systems involved in sexual arousal.

Despite our different external genitals (Illustration 1), males and females are surprisingly similar sexually. However, when it comes to reproduction, we are very different, almost opposite. We start out similarly as foetuses, in a primarily female form. If a Y chromosome is present, then, at around twelve weeks, the seed of the genito-urinary system begins to alter to develop as a male; if not, it continues to develop as female (Bancroft, 1989). A proportion of babies are

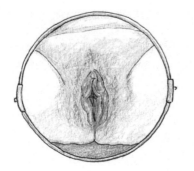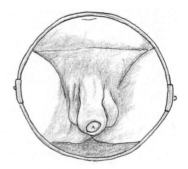

Illustration 1.   External genitals viewed in a mirror.

born with indeterminate genitals; some are allowed to develop until puberty to see what changes emerge and some undergo surgical operations. Our external genitals come in all shapes and sizes, like our different faces. Some adults are also transgendered and might choose to have hormone therapy and/or surgery, which may result in further differences to internal and external sexual organs.

The penis plays a dual role as both a sexual and a reproductive organ for men. Men can be sexual and are potentially fertile all their adult life, from puberty to old age, depending on their health. They can experience sexual pleasure regardless of their fertility: for example, after vasectomy or if infertile through ill health. Men can also experience orgasms, as distinct from their reproductive ability to ejaculate.

Women, however, have separate sexual and reproductive organs, which work independently of each other. Female sexual functioning is separate from reproduction. The monthly menstrual/fertility cycle is not dependent on, or triggered by, sexual activity; it happens regardless of whether women are sexually active or not. Virgins and celibate women still menstruate. Female sexual arousal happens regardless of a woman's ability to conceive; this process is not dependent on, or triggered by, fertility. Women can be sexual at any time but are actually in a physiological infertile state most of their adult life. This is because, between puberty and menopause, women are fertile for only a few days a month, and, during these years, they might have times of being pregnant or breastfeeding. Women can obviously be, and are, sexually potent after menopause.

This is an important awareness, because it demonstrates that our reproductive model of sex is a social construct and not a biological reality. The difference between our reproductive and sexual potential is vital to a new understanding of human sexuality. We can then begin to celebrate our human evolution beyond sex as a reproductive imperative, to see sex also as a socialising and pleasure principle and sexuality as an expression of our fire energy and our creativity.

Exercise   Sensuous skin

Have a bath for the sensuous experience of being in hot water. Prepare the bathroom with candles, bubble bath, or music if you want. Lie for at least fifteen minutes, relax and experience your body, letting the water move on you. What does it feel like, what thoughts and emotions are evoked.

When you get out of the bath, wrap yourself in warm towels, imagine feeling held and snug.

When you are dry, gently massage your body, touching all over your skin. Use lotion or oil if you want. Feel the touch of your skin, how another may experience touching you. What does it feel like inside of you, when you are being touched?

The proud penis

We have a cultural ambivalence towards the penis; a sort of respect for it as a symbol of power and potency with its ability to stand erect, yet a shaming also. Words like dick or prick generally have a social overtone of criticism. Generally, men's clothes include trousers, baggy around the crotch. Men are socially encouraged to hide their sexual attributes, in extreme opposition to those of women, which are emphasised.

Physiology

Even though men and women have different external genitals, there are many internal similarities. The *testes* and *vas deferens* are similar to the ovaries and fallopian tubes in women. The *prostate* and *Cowper's glands* are similar to the uterus and paraurethral glands. The penis is an external equivalent of the internal clitoris. Both have a *glans, shaft,* two *corpus cavernosum,* and the *corpus spongiosum.* Some men have a foreskin and some have had it removed. Illustration 2 shows the internal structure of the flaccid penis within the pelvic area. The dotted lines show how it changes when erect.

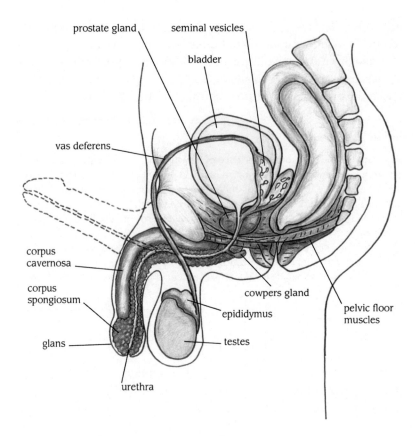

Illustration 2. The internal structure of the penis.

Male fertility

Every day, millions of sperm are made in the *somniferous tubules* in the *testes*. They move into the *epididymus*, learn to swim, and continue up the *vas deferens* to be stored in the *seminal vesicles*. The whole process of sperm production takes about seventy-two days. Because men can manufacture sperm in their bodies, they are potentially fertile all their adult life. The quality of their fertility depends on age, health, and lifestyle.

Arousal

Usually, the shaft of the penis is flaccid and hangs down over the testicles. The penis becomes erect due to changes in the *erectile tissue*:

the corpus cavernosum, the smooth muscle within the penis, changes and blood flows into the corpus spongiosum and swells the shaft. This happens in various stages from first excitation through to full erection. Men do not need a full erection for ejaculation or orgasm. Getting an erection is not always sexual. It is a reflex, an automatic response in the body. Men often wake up with an erection, because the smooth muscle in the penis has relaxed during sleep.

Ejaculation

Ejaculation in males is when semen is released from the penis. Sperm mix with nutrient-rich fluids from the seminal vesicles, the prostate, and Cowper's glands, which is then propelled through the vas deferens and out through the urethral opening at the tip of the penis.

Male orgasm

Orgasm is a reflex action through the nervous system, due to a surge of hormones. It culminates in a release of sexual energy, and pleasurable muscle spasms. Orgasm can be experienced in the genitals, or the whole body can be affected. After orgasm, the body returns to a pre-orgasmic state and can orgasm again and again.

Exercise   External genitals

Bring a small mirror into your safe space, sit for a while and allow yourself to settle. Remove clothes covering your genitals, sit down, and open your legs. Using the mirror, look at your genital area, smile, and say hello. Look in detail at yourself and imagine you have never seen a vulva or penis and scrotum before.

Do a self-portrait or representation of your genitals. It could be a still life or an abstract, a painting, drawing, or a collage.

The wonderful womb

Physiology

Women's reproductive organs are the *ovaries, fallopian tubes, uterus* and the *vagina*. The *vagina* surrounds the tip of the uterus, the *cervix*, providing a birth canal to the entrance within the vulva. Illustration 3

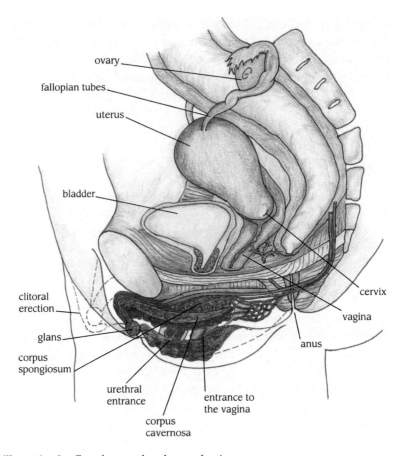

ovary

fallopian tubes

uterus

bladder

clitoral
erection

glans

corpus
spongiosum

urethral
entrance

corpus
cavernosa

entrance to
the vagina

anus

vagina

cervix

Illustration 3.   Female sexual and reproductive organs.

shows the internal structure of the clitoris and the reproductive
organs within the pelvic area. The dotted lines show how the clitoris
changes when erect.

Female fertility

Human females are infertile most of the time, except for a few days
during each monthly cycle. Many women, and men, are not aware of
the menstrual cycle as a fertility cycle. What is actually quite simple—
being aware of this process—is implied as unpredictable, as if women
are somehow *potentially* fertile all the time, so could get pregnant at
any time. Women are born with a limited number of eggs in their

ovaries, making them potentially fertile from menstruation until the menopause. Usually, during each menstrual cycle women ovulate, usually just once. Just as, or soon after, menstruation ends, women begin to become fertile, leading up to ovulation, when an egg is released from the ovary. This egg must be fertilised within twenty-four hours or it disintegrates and is reabsorbed into the body. Fertilisation usually happens in the first part of one of the fallopian tubes. If conception does not happen, the egg will disintegrate and the woman will menstruate again in about two weeks, starting a new fertility cycle.

In the same way that the moon cycles vary between twenty-nine and thirty-one days per month, women's cycles are not always twenty-eight days, but sometimes vary in length. The time from ovulation until the next period is fixed: each woman will have a pattern of between twelve to sixteen days. Once recognised (along with an awareness of when ovulation has occurred), a woman can then accurately predict when her next menstruation will start. Some months might be a shorter cycle and some a longer cycle. This is because the day of ovulation can vary in each cycle, but it will always be preceded with the signs of fertility outlined below. By observing and charting changes in both the cervix and the cervical fluid, woman can get to know what their body is like when it is infertile: the "basic infertile pattern", and how it changes during the few fertile days.

The basic infertile pattern of the cervix is that it protrudes into the vagina and can be felt by inserting one or two fingers; it will feel easy to reach and relatively firm. During each cycle, the cervix goes through changes similar to that of the birthing process; it softens and shortens in increments, so that just before ovulation it can feel higher up in the vagina and more difficult to reach, and the os, the opening to the cervix, has changed from being closed to more open. This may take several days to happen. After ovulation, it returns to its infertile state of feeling firmer and lower in the vagina. In conjunction with these changes, glands in the cervix produce fluids, which change over several days building up to the day of ovulation, and then also change again after.

It is easiest to think of the first day of a menstrual bleed as the beginning of a new cycle, and of each cycle having three phases.

1. The first phase of these changes is called the *potentially fertile phase* because we are infertile until our fertility begins, which we

cannot predict but need to observe cycle by cycle. Following the menstrual period, there might be several days of no visible fluids; these days may be absent in short cycles and numerous in long cycles.

2.   One of the first signs of the *fertile phase* is a sensation or presentation of a moist or sticky fluid in the vagina; it is usually scant, pasty, and white or yellow in colour. There is then a transitional stage where increasing amounts of slightly stretchy, cloudy, and thinner fluids may be felt or observed. Highly fertile fluids will become more profuse, giving a sensation of lubrication or slipperiness. The appearance will be thin, watery, and transparent, and, at its peak, stretchy and similar to raw egg white. Ovulation happens just after the peak of these changes.

3.   During the *post-ovulatory phase*, the slippery sensation is lost and there will be a relatively abrupt return to stickiness or dryness again; the cervical fluids have thickened again, forming a plug at the cervix, acting as a barrier to sperm, and reducing the chances of infection within the reproductive organs. As the amount and quality of these fluids will vary from woman to woman, charting to get to know her "basic infertile pattern" is the best way for each woman to understand her patterns in the signs of fertility.

Cervical fluids can be distinguished from semen or arousal lubrication; the latter two will dry up quickly upon your fingertips and are water soluble. If confused, test the fluid by dipping it into a glass of water. If it is fertile cervical fluid, it will form a ball and sink to the bottom, if not, it will dissolve. Cervical fluids are crucial to fertility, playing several roles, including filtering out any damaged sperm. Ordinarily, sperm would die within a few hours after ejaculation, but in this fertile fluid, they can live for up to five days, occasionally longer. What is clinically called "discharge" is actually an alkaline "sperm- friendly" fluid, providing channels to help them swim the long distance. If the sperm reach a fertile egg, they will be able to fuse with it, having been chemically activated and stripped of their outer coating of zinc and proteins by the cervical fluid. Understanding the cyclical changes in fluids can help women to know when something is not right and can encourage early detection of a sexually transmitted infection or other gynaecological difficulty.

Other indicators of the ovulatory process include changes in body temperature, breast tenderness, and sometimes a sharp twinge in the ovary concerned. The body temperature is lower before ovulation and higher afterwards; charting this will show the differences. This is useful to indicate that ovulation has happened, but not helpful in indicating the onset of the fertile phase. Women's *fertile phase* is about five days before ovulation, because of the cervical fluids, and for twenty-four hours after.

Exercise   First reproductive experience

What are your first thoughts when you think about your *first menstruation* or your *first wet dream*? Had you been informed about the biology of what was happening? Were there any adults around to explain things to you?

How did you feel? Were there any surprises, and, if so, what were they?

What do you think and how do you feel now thinking about this time?

The voluptuous vulva

We have a cultural dislike for women's external genitals, which is called the *vulva*. It is actually confusing that we distinguish the clitoris and the vulva. It probably came about because of the reproductive model of sex: the focus on the vagina as women's sexual organ, and a need to name and identify women's external sexual genitalia. It was like talking about our throat and pretending we do not have a mouth, tongue, or lips. By ignoring the vulva, we miss out what is within it, the clitoris, which, as you will see in the next section, is not a "tiny, hard to find bud". There are many other colloquial words, such as fanny, pussy, and cunt, which do refer to the whole vulva. Despite being reclaimed by some, the word cunt is still the most offensive swearword we have.

Physiology

The vulva is the oval area, with all its different parts and shapes; it is the outside part of women's sexual organ, the *clitoris*. Most of the clitoris and the vagina are inside the body. When the lips of the vulva are open, we can see the glans of the clitoris and the entrance to the vagina. The vagina leads from the opening in the vulva up to the cervix, the end part of the uterus (Illustration 4).

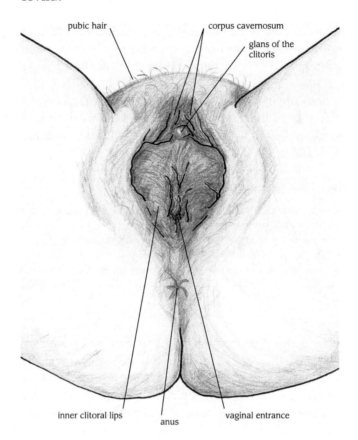

pubic hair

corpus cavernosum

glans of the
clitoris

inner clitoral lips

anus

vaginal entrance

Illustration 4.   The open vulva.

Exercise   Genital geography

Bring a small mirror into your safe space, sit for a while and allow yourself to settle. Remove clothes covering your genitals, sit down, and open your legs. Using the mirror, look at your genital area, smile, and say hello. Look in detail at yourself.

Gently touch and explore to see all the aspects of your genitals. For those with penises, include the shaft and the tip, move the foreskin back, feel your testicles. For those with vulvas, touch all the outside areas and then open the inner vulva lips and feel the different parts and places, including inside the vagina. Then afterwards, explore the perineum and your anus.

What it is like to touch and be touched. Smell and taste your fingers when touching different parts of yourself. Notice any sensations in your body and any feelings evoked.

Using the pictures in this book, see if you can map out your unique genital geography. Notice different shapes, colours, and textures. Can you identify all the different aspects of your genitals?

What do you call your genitals: vulva, fanny, pussy, cunt, penis, dick, cock, or prick? What do you like to say, what do you like to hear?

The cunning clitoris

In our culture, we cut out women's sexual organs visually and linguistically; in other cultures, this is done literally. The Prohibition of Female Circumcision Act came into force in the UK in 1985, making it an offence to carry out, or to aid or procure the performance by another person, of any form of female genital mutilation (FGM), except for specific medical purpose. Estimates show that around 66,000 women resident in England and Wales have been subjected to FGM. In 2004, there were around 30,500 estimated numbers of maternities in England and Wales in women likely to have undergone FGM (End Violence Against Women, 2007).

Physiology

Women's sexual organs include the *clitoris*, which is as wide and as long as the vulva, from the *pubic bone* to the *anus*. The erectile tissue of the clitoris, the *glans*, two *corpus cavernosum*, and the *corpus spongiosum* also extends inside the body, surrounding the *entrance to the vagina*. Two excellent books with details about the clitoris are *A New View of a Woman's Body* (Federation of Feminist Women's Health Centers (FFWHC), 1995) and *The Clitoral Truth* (Chalker, 2000). Illustration 5 shows the internal structure of the clitoris.

Illustration 6 shows the outline of the external vulva, so you can see the clitoral system as it is internally. This shows clearly that the vulva is women's primary sexual organ. There is sexual sensitivity in the first third of the vagina, as it is surrounded by the corpus spongiosum, the erectile tissue of the clitoris.

Arousal

The *clitoral bud* is similar to the very tip of the penis. When it is erect, the whole clitoris is actually thirty times bigger than the little bud.

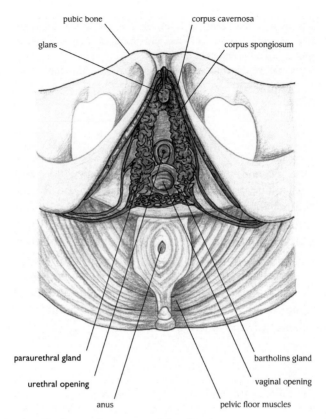

Illustration 5. The internal structure of the clitoris.

There are two *bartholins glands*, one on each side of the vaginal opening. When women are sexually aroused, fluids are produced from these glands, which make the vulva feel wet. The *perineal sponge*, between the vaginal entrance and the anus, is also sexually sensitive. The *pelvic floor muscles* play a crucial role in the sexual arousal process, in both men and women, particularly at orgasm.

Ejaculation

The clitoris also surrounds the urethra, creating the *urethral sponge*, or *G zone*, as it is more commonly called. Stimulation of this area can lead to female ejaculate being released from the *paraurethral glands*. Analysis has shown that fluids released by women are the same as male ejaculate, but without any sperm (FFWHC, 1995).

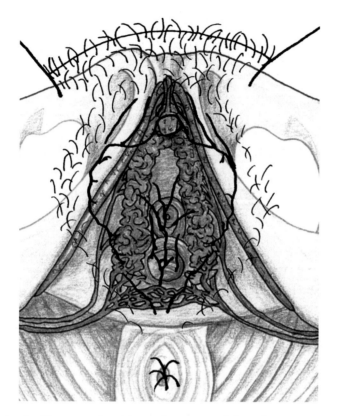

Illustration 6.   The external and internal structure of the vulva.

Female orgasm

Orgasm is a reflex action through the nervous system, due to a surge of hormones. It culminates in a release of sexual energy, and pleasurable muscle spasms. Orgasm can be experienced in the genitals, or the whole body can be affected. After orgasm, the body returns to a pre-orgasmic state and can orgasm again and again.

Exercise   Tender touch

Make a time for yourself in your safe space. Make it warm. Take your clothes off, sit for a few moments, and settle. Close your eyes and put your hands on your face. Touch your face, forehead, cheeks, and chin. Feel your skin being touched. Touch your neck shoulders and both arms.

Experiment with your touch; firmer, softer, slow and fast, longer strokes or circles. Touch with your fingers, palms, back of your hand. Try kisses with lips and tongues. Explore and touch your feet, toes, legs, and torso, but for this exercise do not touch your nipples, breasts, genitals, or anus. Notice what touch you like where, why, and how. What turns you on?

What ideas, desires, thoughts, and imaginations are triggered?

Do you want to go with the flow and want to become sexual? Have you cut off, numbed at the thought of any particular memories or emotions? If so, notice what has turned you off. Maybe it's thoughts or beliefs that might be outmoded now. Remember to "apply the brakes" if necessary.

Reflect on this experience and either talk with someone, write, or draw.

Outside in

Having described the sexual organs and their arousal process, we can now consider other changes in the body during sexual arousal. Another obvious erogenous area is the breasts and nipples in both men and women. Sexual arousal brings a heightened sensitivity and changes in shape and colour to these areas. It also causes changes to our breathing patterns, muscle tension and blood flow, hormone circulation and activity, and a heightening of the nervous system.

Our various senses are like a gateway through which we experience the outside world, other people, and our environment. We might see or hear something, which then passes through the sensory nerve pathways to the brain, where the stimulus will be assessed via our memory centres and then responded to, all in seconds. Our sensuality includes the five senses of sight, smell, touch, taste, and sound (Figure 5), and our sensuality is a precursor to sexuality. We can think about each of the senses in turn and contemplate what we enjoy and what we do not. For example, if you think about the sense of smell, which aromas are pleasing to you, which turn you on, and which turn you off? The same can be considered for each of the other senses: sight, touch, taste, and sound. What pleases us is unique to each individual.

But what exactly is sexual arousal? First, let us consider the word arousal. As humans, we are constantly reacting and responding to stimuli from our outside world. These stimuli trigger a range of automatic, internal responses, most of which are happening so fast and so unconsciously that we do not even notice. As explained earlier, we are reacting with our brain, our beliefs, our bodies, and our feelings, all affecting and being affected by the others.

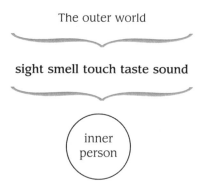

The outer world

sight smell touch taste sound

inner
person

Figure 5.   The five senses.

Our whole body is activated during sexual arousal, and feeling sensations and energy specifically in our genitals is an indication of feeling sexually aroused, as opposed to other types of arousal. We can consider that our body is not feeling, say, hunger, until we experience a trigger to arousal, which might be an inner sensation of our belly grumbling or an outer awareness, such as seeing or smelling food we like. We will discuss triggers to sexual arousal later.

Feeling stimulated into a sexual charge is not that different than, say, feeling hungry, or the urge to shout or cry. There will be an automatic physical response, an energy charge in the body, which sometimes we react to unconsciously, and at other times we make daily decisions and choices about. For example, even though we might feel angry and experience an urge or a desire to shout at someone, we might decide it is inappropriate or not wise to do so. The point is that even though we feel something, we do not always act on that feeling. As described in Part I about the mind and our belief systems, we humans are very capable of controlling or suppressing any feelings.

Exercise   Sensuality

Take your attention to your sense of *sight*. Think about sights, visions, and images that turn you *on*, make you feel good. Now think about what turns you *off*. How does that make you feel? Notice what happens in your body to your breath, heartbeat, and your muscles. Notice your thoughts.

Take your attention to your sense of *sound*. What sounds do you like, what turns you *on*, makes you feel good? Now think about what turns you *off*. How does that make you feel? Notice what happens in your body, to your breath, heartbeat, and muscles. Notice your thoughts.

Now think about your sense of *smell*. What smells turn you *on*? Now think about what turns you *off*. How does that make you feel? Notice what happens in your body, to your breath, heartbeat, and muscles. Notice your thoughts.

What about your sense of *taste*? What tastes do you like? What tastes turn you *on* and which turn you *off*? How does that make you feel? Notice what happens in your body, to your breath, heartbeat, and muscles. Notice your thoughts.

Now think about your sense of *touch*. What things that you touch turn you *on*? In what ways do you like to be touched, where and how, what sort of pressure? Now think about what turns you *off*. How does that make you feel? Notice what happens in your body, to your breath, heartbeat, and muscles. Notice your thoughts.

Want somebody

Our reproductive model of sex encourages us to focus on the genitals and not pay much attention to other parts of our body involved in sexual response. Inside our skin we have a skeleton of bones, surrounded by muscles and tissue and many vital and secondary organs. Our heart pumps blood and hormones around the body and our lungs and respiratory system oxygenate and mobilise our body. Sexual arousal causes changes to our muscles and our breathing patterns, triggered by hormonal activity, and a heightening of the sensitivity of our nervous system.

Of the five senses, touch is a vital aspect of our sexuality, both touching and being touched. It is through our skin that we experience touching and being touched, an activity which stimulates feel-good hormones such as oxytocin (Odent, 1999; Panksepp, 1998). Our skin is the largest body organ; it is what keeps all our organs and body systems inside our body and it marks a boundary between us each as individual human beings, and the outer world of our environment and other people. Our whole skin is an erogenous zone, with highly sensitive nerve endings, but especially our fingertips, genitals, and lips. The desire to kiss, to touch, and make contact with another's lips is another indicator of sexual arousal.

With sexual arousal, we often experience a desire to reach out and make contact with another, to touch both literally and metaphorically. This desire for other is an important awareness in a new understanding of sexuality, as it reminds us about the relational connections. Primarily, we want someone, not something; our urge is for an "other" to share with sexually.

In our model of sex as an act, we talk about making love to someone, not with them; we objectify our sexuality. Thinking in a new way
about sex and sexuality, in a more wholistic and integrative way,
we can encourage a more subjective experience, as we will explore in
this book. We can think about being sexual to mean expressing our
sexuality in many ways, maybe including behaving sexually and
maybe not. We can consider and evaluate, and then choose how we
act.

Exercise   Body and breath awareness

Take yourself to your safe space when you have at least thirty minutes to spare
and when you will not be disturbed. Get yourself into a really comfortable and
warm sitting or lying position. Close your eyes and allow a few minutes to settle
and begin to relax. Notice sounds around you, and just let them be; notice the
thoughts you have and let them go.

Focus on your out-breath; imagine you are gently blowing out through a straw,
then just allow the in-breath to follow. Do this for a while until you feel your
body relaxing. Notice your thoughts, then just allow them to pass.

Scan down your body and imagine any tensions leaving with the out-breath;
from your forehead, your eyes and jaw; your neck muscles, shoulders, arms and
hands; down your back, across your chest, your stomach, and pelvis; your genitals and buttocks, legs, ankles, and feet.

For a while, allow yourself to just sit or lie and focus on the rhythmic pattern
of your breath coming in and leaving, just noticing and being aware of your body.
If you become distracted, don't worry, just take your attention back to your
breathing.

Place one hand on your heart and one hand on your genitals and continue to
focus on your out-breath then your in-breath. Notice any changes since you have
done this. Just sit for a few minutes to get a sense of a connection between these
two parts of your body.

When you are ready to complete this relaxation, first consciously deepen your
breathing and become more mindful of where you are before you open your eyes.
Stretch if you want, and wiggle your fingers and toes.

Sit quietly for a few moments and reflect on your experience. You may want
to write or draw a picture about it.

Happy hormones

During sexual arousal, all of the body systems are involved in a
network of communication, between our bodies and our brains, via
the *endocrine* and the *nervous systems*. Neurochemicals are made in the

brain and can be distributed throughout the whole body through the nervous system. These chemicals can also be transformed into hormones and be directed to specific organs or areas of the body by the endocrine system. Hormones travel via the blood stream.

The main endocrine gland is the pituitary, which regulates the activities of this system. The other glands include the thyroid, which regulates growth and metabolism, the pancreas, which regulates digestion and insulin, the adrenal gland, which produces hormones for survival, such as fight and flight, and the ovaries and testes, which regulate reproduction.

When we take in the outside world through our senses, it stimulates the hypothalamus in the brain, which activates the endocrine and nervous system. The release of hormones sets off a chain of events, affecting many body systems. Hormones include endorphins and opiates, which are natural painkillers. They are our own free, natural "feel good" chemicals, which induce pleasurable emotions and sensations, with no come-downs or side-effects. The hormones involved in the sexual arousal process are, not surprisingly, similar to those involved in fertility and birthing (Kitzinger, 1985) (Figure 6). One of them, oxytocin, is known as the bonding hormone and is sometimes called the "love drug"; it pulses rhythmically through the body during sexual arousal and birthing. There is then a surge and a peak at orgasm, just as there is at the moment of delivery. Oxytocin also triggers the orgasmic reflex.

Exercise   Your delights and pleasures

Think about something general that gives you pleasure. Notice how it feels inside your body: what physical sensations and emotional reactions are triggered. Notice what thoughts are generated.

Now think about something that pleases you sexually, and again notice the sensations, emotions, and thoughts. Spend more time considering your different senses (sights, sounds, smells, tastes, ways of touching and being touched) that arouse you, until you feel really familiar with what feeling pleasure feels like physically and emotionally.

Turn your attention to your imagination. Give yourself at least ten minutes; allow yourself to wander and dream, to see what images come into your mind triggered by you delighting in your senses. Which senses are most pleasurable to you? How do they make you feel physically and emotionally?

Sex hormones	Effects
DHEA Dehydroepiandosterone	master sex hormone, increases desire, boosts energy and reduces stress
Androstenedione	increases testosterone, enhances libido
Estrogen and Testosterone	control fertility, motivate sexual interest, increase Oxytocin
Adrenaline	alertness, fires up energy, increases heart beat
Prostaglandins	contract smooth muscle in genitals, stimulate and sharpen senses
Acetylcholine	relaxation, parasympathetic nervous system
Pheromones	scents we secrete which excite us and attract others
Endorphins and Opiates	natural pain killers, relaxants, stimulated by play and touch
Oxytocin	relaxation, empathy, bonding and attachment, peaks at orgasm

Figure 6.   Sex hormones and their effects.

The nervous system

The sexual arousal charge moves through the parasympathetic branch of the autonomic nervous system to cause genital arousal and the sympathetic branch is activated for ejaculation and for orgasm. Sexual arousal may be triggered by an outside stimulus via the senses, or by an emotion or an internal body sensation. It can also be activated by the imagination or by a memory. All will feed back to the brain, which will activate the autonomic nervous system to react as described above. There are many nerve rich areas in the human body. The most pronounced are the lips, the fingertips, and the genitals. Illustrations 7 and 8 show the nerves in the female and male pelvis.

The nervous system plays a central role in the sexual arousal process sending neurotransmitters (brain chemicals) throughout the body. It has different elements: the *central nervous system* (the CNS), which is the brain and spinal cord and the *peripheral nervous system*, (the PNS) (Figure 7). The PNS relays information to and from the

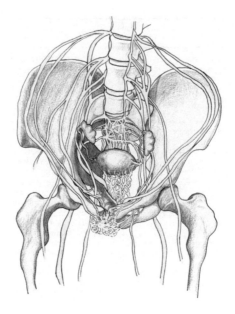

Illustration 7.   Female pelvic nerves.

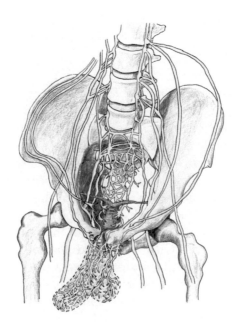

Illustration 8.   Male pelvic nerves.

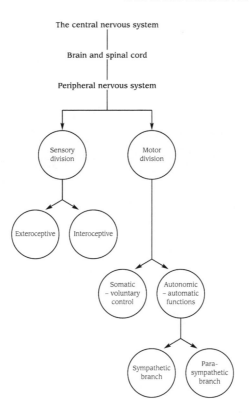

The central nervous system

Brain and spinal cord

Peripheral nervous system

Sensory division

Motor division

Exteroceptive

Interoceptive

Somatic – voluntary control

Autonomic – automatic functions

Sympathetic branch

Para-sympathetic branch

Figure 7. The nervous system.

body, and to and from the CNS. It has two aspects: the *sensory division* and the *motor division*. The sensory division also has two aspects. The *exteroceptive* includes our five senses, sight, sound, touch, taste, and smell, which take the outside world in. The *interoceptive* includes the internal experience of our body organs, such as pain and proprioception, the relationship of the body internally, of various body parts to others.

The motor division also has two parts: somatic and autonomic. *Somatic* nerves control conscious functions, like moving muscles and *autonomic* nerves control reflexes, the automatic reactions, such as breathing and heart rate. The autonomic nervous system also has two parts. Essentially, our bodies are either relaxed or activated into arousal. The *sympathetic* nervous system moves us into arousal and the *parasympathetic* takes us back into relaxation. The genital area is dense with nerves, to the clitoris in women and to the penis and prostate gland in men.

Another nerve worth mentioning is the vagus, which meanders through the body with branches connecting with the abdomen, heart, lungs, stomach, and ears, among other body parts. It carries incoming information from the nervous system to the brain, providing information about what the body is doing. It also transmits outgoing information that governs a range of reflex responses, including our breathing, heartbeat, and muscle control. Recent research by Komisaruk, Beyer-Flores, and Whipple, 2006 has also shown four different nerve pathways via the vagus nerve that carry sensory signals from the vagina, cervix, clitoris, and uterus, which can all contribute to orgasms. It is believed that people with spinal cord injury are able to experience orgasm via the vagus nerve, which travels outside the spinal cord and into the brain. They have also documented in the laboratory that women can have orgasms from imagery alone, without touching their bodies, and that women can experience orgasms and sexual pleasure from many more forms of stimuli than stimulation of the genitals.

So far we have explored our thoughts, beliefs, and values about sex and sexuality in the section titled "Mind". In this section, the Body, we have described in detail the anatomy and physiology of sexual arousal, separating our reproductive functioning and our sexual arousal process. We have discussed the biology of sex, including not just the genital changes but also how our respiratory system and musculature is affected. We can see how the changes are activated through the endocrine system transporting hormones and the nervous system in relaying messages between our bodies and our brains.

We have seen the relationships between ourselves and others; our inner and outer worlds, the pairs within our nervous system, and our interrelating within the body through feedback loops. The relational desire in the sexual urge to reach out, to touch an "other", could inspire us to see sex as more than an act that someone does. We can begin to value our sexuality as something more complex and integrated, more subjective and experiential. In the next section, we will discuss another element of our sexual experiences, the brain, and explore the neurochemistry and stages of sexual arousal and the interrelatedness between our thinking, our bodies, and our brains.

Exercise   Review of Part II

Read back through the exercises for this section and what you have written in your journal. Take some time to reflect on your exploration and to evaluate your work. Which exercises did you like and which ones did you not like? Think about why.

What have you discovered about your body and your sensuality? Have any discoveries surprised you? If so, what and why? How do you feel about this?

What have you discovered about your sexual arousal? Does it differ if you do this exercise at different times and in difference places: if so, which do you prefer?

Are there any exercises that you would like to do again? If so, notice what is similar or different if you do them a second time.

Is there anything you want to change? If so, how could you do that?

Talk to someone, write or draw something about how you are thinking and feeling having worked on this section.

PART III

BRAIN: PASSION AND DESIRE

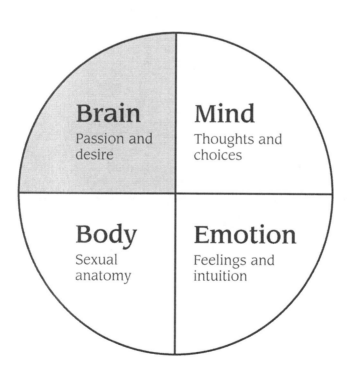

Brain, mind, body, and emotion.

The brain

Frisson

I n this section, we will explore the brain in more detail with regard to sexuality and sexual functioning. It is often said we cannot help whom we fall in love with, which has some truth in it. Day by day, we are having instant reactions, which we are constantly evaluating and choosing to act on, or not. By describing in more detail what happens physiologically in the brain, we can gain a deeper under-standing of why we experience our sexuality as we do as humans. We can also begin to comprehend how our brain interacts with our minds and our bodies, as described in the previous sections, giving us a clearer idea of why we react as we do and why we choose to behave in some ways and not in others.

So, what is it that happens in that moment when someone catches our eye and triggers our interest in them? Research about sexual attraction is inconclusive, except that when an attraction happens, it will be registered within seconds. We will explore in more depth the instinctual reactions and reflexes of the brain, in particular the limbic system, sometimes called the "social brain" or the seat of our emotions.

Sexual interest has an impact on all aspects of us, as described in this interactive model for sexuality. In our mind, our frontal lobes, we can become preoccupied with thoughts and choices about how we could make things happen. Our imagination can begin to run wild with potentials and possibilities. We will also be aware of our social and cultural beliefs, which might encourage our desires or present prohibitions.

Sexual arousal neurochemicals are triggered in the inner regions of the brain and our memory centres are activated. There can be many changes in the body, including an increase in our heartbeat, body temperature, and breathing rate, a tightness in the stomach, and a stirring in the genitals. There will be a heightened arousal of all our senses and the nervous system. Many feelings and emotions will be stirring, and this is all in the first five minutes. An interactive chain of events has been initiated in our inner world by a stimulus of something or someone in our internal world or from the outer world. The sexual arousal circuit has been activated, been turned on.

Morin (1996) has provided much insight into our relationship with the erotic through his research. He suggests that by reviewing our "peak erotic experiences" and discovering exactly what made them so, we can discover our "core erotic theme": our internal blueprint for arousal. He offers a sexual excitement survey and suggests ways to explore your unique erotic fingerprint. This can be useful where there are any difficulties with low sexual desire, or to enhance your relationship to your erotic desire.

Exercise   Desire

Think about your desire. Write about what this word means for you. How does desire differ from "want" or "need"?

Write a list of your desires, generally. Write a list of your sexual desires.

Take some time to review what you have written and notice what you think and feel about what you have written. Do your desires sit comfortably with your beliefs and values? If not, do you wish to re-evaluate your desires, and/or your beliefs and values?

The busy brain

Historically, most research on the brain was conducted on people with injury; our knowledge about brain functioning was extrapolated from how damage to certain areas was seen to affect behaviours. With the advent of technology to see inside our brains, we now know that certain areas are activated and "light up" during different activities. We understand more about sexual neurochemistry and the role of our brain in sexual functioning.

We know more about the distinctions and relationship between the frontal "thinking" lobes and the deeper, more primitive reflexive areas. The *brain stem* is one of the most primal aspects of the brain, and includes the *medulla oblongata*, which regulates reflexes such as heart rate, blood flow, and breathing, all affected during sexual arousal (Illustration 9). The brain is continually evaluating triggers from the outside world and the inner body, and is continually responding to these stimuli. In nanoseconds, decisions are being made with us being in a state of constant interaction—homeodynamic function, as described earlier.

The *cerebellum* controls and co-ordinates movement and the *cerebrum* receives the messages from our senses, such as sight and sound.

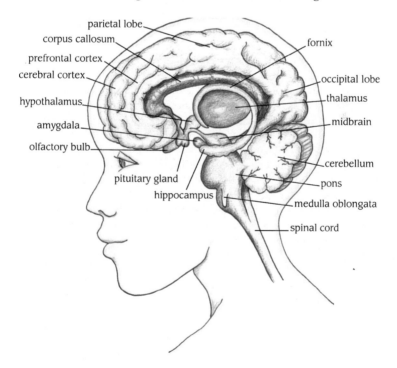

Illustration 9. The brain.

Other areas in the brain are primary centres for speech and learning, and the frontal lobes are considered to oversee personality and intelligence. The more we learn about the brain, the more we realise how complex, interactive, and interrelational all elements are. Deep with the brain sits a cluster of cells and systems referred to as the limbic system, a crucial element in sexual functioning.

Exercise   Emotional awareness I

Take some time to sit and relax. Allow your body, your breath, and your heartbeat to settle. Remember a time when you felt sad. Notice your body: where do you feel sadness? Notice any muscle tension or discomfort. Now notice what sort of memories come to mind. What is your internal dialogue about these memories? Spend a few moments with your experiences about sadness, then take some deep breaths and allow your thoughts and feelings to pass.

Now take your attention to the emotion of fear. Again, notice first what happens in your body: where do you feel fear somatically? What is happening to your breath and your heartbeat? Notice your memories and your thoughts and what you are thinking about, what you are experiencing. Allow some time to be with what is happening and then imagine just letting it go. You might want to imagine breathing out through a straw, long, slow breaths.

Repeat this exercise thinking about anger, noticing your body and becoming familiar with the sensations, thoughts, and beliefs you have when experiencing the emotion of anger.

Now turn your attention to feelings of joy and happiness, and what sensations then happen in your body. How is your breathing and heartbeat now? What memories are evoked, and what sort of mind talk is happening? Stay with these feelings longer than with the others, and revel in feeling joy.

Write or reflect on the similarities and differences of how you experience each of these emotions in your body and what impact they have on your breathing and your heart rate. Notice what you were thinking about each of them. Which emotions do you feel comfortable with and which do you not?

How were emotions dealt with in your family? Were certain feelings encouraged and others disallowed? Reflect on what you have written about your relationships to your emotions now and how this may correlate with your childhood experiences.

The limbic system

The limbic system is the name given to a group of brain structures including the hypothalamus, the thalamus, the hippocampus, and the amygdala. The hypothalamus regulates our urges and appetites, acting as a bridge between our brain and our body. It directs the thalamus as to which neurochemicals it should release, in which quantities, and when. The amygdala and hippocampus systems are part of our memory centre. All internal and external stimuli are evaluated primarily by our memory centres; it is our first port of call: do I know this, have I experienced this before? As infants, we learn through memory; we store experiences in our memory centres to draw on as we need. We are continually building our story of the world and how it works.

The hippocampus also connects with an area called the periaqueductal grey (PAG), which registers our experiences of pain and pleasure. The amygdala stores the raw experience and the hippocampus orders the time sequence of events. The amygdala can be seen to act as an alarm system, alerting us to the need for fight or flight. For example, if we suddenly hear a loud noise, the sound might be stored in our memory as, say, a car back-firing: we register that we know what it is, and react or ignore it. If we do not know what it is, we might look to see; again we might remember what this is and, again, react or ignore.

Recent research has taught us much about how trauma affects the limbic system, particularly. Our emotional centre can become overwhelmed in responses to certain stimuli; we are literally flooded with neurochemicals as the amygdala triggers an alert. Survival circuits become activated; there could be horrific images and incidences, experiences stored in the memory centres. We might go into rage, disassociation, or a state of freeze, like a rabbit in headlights. If our brain circuits have been over-activated in childhood, neural pathways can become "hardwired", leading to a heightened reactivity to, and propensity for, fear or rage.

Studies into post traumatic stress disorder have shown damage to the hippocampus. It seems that when people suffer flashbacks, for example, feelings, sensations, and memories are experienced as if they are happening now, rather than as events from the past, as if the time sequencing has gone askew. It is uncertain whether the traumatic event caused the damage, or whether the person is suffering post trauma because their hippocampus was already faulty.

Trauma is an important consideration concerning sexual issues, because many people have experienced sexualised violence as children and/or as adults. It can affect our brains, bodies, hearts, and minds and will be discussed in a wider context in the next section. Herman (1993) widened our understanding of trauma, to include all forms of emotional, sexual, and physical violence, specifically within a powerless environment. She also believed it vital that recovery should occur within a healing and safe relationship. Touch and sensory experiences are central to our sexuality; they can also trigger traumatic memory. Our emotions hold memories, as do our bodies. Pert (1998) has shown there are neurotransmitter receptor sites not just in the brain, but throughout the body, indicating the physiology of the brain–body feedback loops. Therapists such as Levine (1997) and Rothschild (2000) have contributed great understanding to the theory and treatment of post trauma stress, combining our knowledge from neuroscience and body psychotherapy. Recovery is focused on soothing the arousal circuits in the brain, body, emotions, and thinking processes.

We can also be reactive to many things that we would not necessarily consider to be traumatic; they can just be issues or incidences that did have an impact on our limbic system in our past and still activate us now. Some people get hot under the collar about things that other people seem to take in their stride, such as injustice or being disbelieved, for example. Some find themselves furious if people cancel appointments or are late, others take it in their stride; some hate being ignored, while others might not notice. We could take this as information to understand ourselves better and to realise that where there is heat, there is history. If we find ourselves somewhat over reactive to something, we could explore why and find out what might be underlying our reaction.

Exercise   Triggers

Take some time to think about what sort of events or situations you know you react to in comparison to how you see others react. Choose one to explore in more depth.

Write in detail about an incident that happened recently and include how you felt. Notice your body sensations as well as emotions and thoughts. See if you can identify exactly what it was that upset you. If you find this difficult, imagine what you would have liked to have happened differently.

Think back to your childhood and see if you can remember whether this was something that used to happen to you then. Write about how you felt then and consider how familiar your feelings were then to how they are now.

Explore whether there are other feelings behind the ones you usually feel or express. Consider what it would be like to express these feelings instead.

Brain chemicals

There are many brain chemicals, called neurotransmitters, that affect human sexuality. They are released from the inner regions of the brain, the limbic system, to the central nervous system, and then flood through the body through the peripheral nervous system. As nerves pass these chemical messages to each other, links and pathways are created that run quicker and quicker the more they are used. Like learning to play an instrument, the more we practise the easier it becomes. We become conditioned, which is partly how we learn.

Neurochemicals can also be transformed via the hypothalamus to become hormones, which are then sent through the bloodstream, usually to a specific place in the body, whereas neurotransmitters pass through the nervous system to many areas. These substances are made in the brain and affected by our diet. A healthy diet will ensure a good supply of those needed for emotional well-being in the same way that a diet balanced in proteins, carbohydrates, vitamins, and minerals will support our physical health. Equally, a diet depleted in nutrients such as vitamins and minerals will undermine our mental health and ability to deal with the everyday stresses in life.

The main brain chemicals involved in the sexual arousal process and their functions are:

- dopamine—motivation, curiosity, intensifies pleasure;
- serotonin—arousal, joy, excitement;
- vasopressin—stimulates genital erection;
- noradrenalin—increases sexual arousal and stimulation;
- endorphins —natural painkillers, relaxants, and opiates, stimulated by play and touch;
- acetylcholine—is stabilised by comfort and soothing;
- oxytocin—relaxation, empathy, bonding, and attachment, peaks at orgasm, triggered by touch;
- phenyl ethylamine (PEA)—the euphoria of "falling in love", affects digestion and the heart (Crenshaw, 1997).

Some of these neurochemicals are known these days in relationship to what people know about recreational drugs. Alcohol activates GABA, a brain chemical that regulates anxiety levels; taking Ecstasy results in more serotonin in the body, which heightens arousal, attention, and excitement, and dopamine, which triggers motivation and initiating action. Noradrenalin pathways are stimulated by Ritalin, cocaine, speed and amphetamines. Some, such as acetychloine, can have varying impacts: separation distress triggers high levels in the brain, whereas in the body it can have a calming effect, activating the parasympathetic nervous system.

Sexual activity triggers many of these feel-good chemicals and can lead to compulsivity and, in some cases, addiction. A recent article (Kessler, 2010) highlighted how some in the food industry are cynically using our knowledge of the body's reward system to create an optimum sugar, fat, and salt combination which triggers dopamine and makes us want to eat more. Whether our current model of sex is equivalent to a type of "fast food", with its own range of health concerns, is a question addressed further in the next section.

Exercise   Feel good

Think about a recent time when you felt really happy and joyous. Spend time recalling where you were, who you were with, and what was being said or done, what was happening. Go over the details and revel in remembering your experience.

Take your attention to your body. Where are you feeling your happiness, in which parts of your body and in what way? Try to imagine the feel good hormones being pumped from your brain through your body into your nervous system, your muscles, and organs. Notice your breathing and your heartbeat. Become really aware of what it feels like physically to feel happy.

Notice your thoughts; are other memories of similar scenarios being evoked? There might be some sadness about the fact that people or times in your history are no longer with you. If so, leave this aside for the moment, and focus back on your joy. How easy is it for you to do this?

Notice what sort of dialogue you have with yourself while you're happy: what types of words, what tone and pitch of voice? How does this differ from when you feel sad, scared, or angry?

Take some time to write about what you have experienced and then to reflect on what you have written.

Human universals

We have been discussing our reactivity and instinctual reactions to understand what they are; whether we are slave to them and how much conscious control we can exert. We have discussed our physiological responses to the directives of neurotransmitters and hormones from the brain in response to triggers. We have acknowledged the role of our frontal lobes, our thinking capacity to make choices in nanoseconds. We are all making thousands of different decisions every day, dependent on our different histories, where we are on the globe, our cultures and customs. So, what is universal, innate in, and to, all of us?

In the 1970s, Ekman's anthropological study of peoples who had previously been socially isolated found they could recognise six human facial expressions (Ekman, 1980). Since then we have believed this was regardless of culture or geography, displayed by all and recognisable in others. In 2009, Callaway's study with East Asian and Caucasians to interpret a standardised set of facial expressions about fear and disgust indicated that they might not be universally applicable, but culturally nuanced.

Tomkins expanded on the notion of primary feelings and the six universally recognised facial expressions. He described what he called "affects", in that they are feelings, triggered by something or someone, that have an impact on our body, causing physical sensations and are visibly recognisable by specific body postures and facial expressions (Kaufman & Raphael, 1996). These eight affects can be experienced ranging from low intensity to high intensity, and are culturally valued as positive, neutral, or negative.

The emotion of happiness is seen to range from *enjoying yourself*, from being pleased, satisfied, and contented to *joyful* (feeling glad, ecstatic, walking on air). The affect is seen in a smile, where the lips widen up and out. He also added the notion of excitement, ranging from mildly *interested* (being curious, fascinated, intrigued, to the more intense feeling of being *excited* (thrilled, eager, or happy). Here, the eyebrows are down and the eyes track, look, and watch. The sex drive is believed to derive its power from the affect of excitement. *Surprise* is seen as a neutral affect, from feeling amazed, astonished, impressed, through to the more intense experience of being *startled* (jolted, shocked, or alarmed). The eyebrows arch, the eyes open wide and blink, and the jaw drops slightly.

The emotions of anger, fear, and sadness, are labelled as negative, perhaps because we know they cause us to feel distress. Being *angry* (irritated, indignant, or resentful), or *enraged* (furious, "seeing red"), are recognised by the eyebrows being lowered, a frown, lips pressed firmly in, a clenched jaw, and sometimes a red face. Being *fearful*:

scared, frightened, nervous, or *terrified* (petrified, in a panic) will show as the eyebrows being raised, eyes frozen open, the mouth slightly open, facial trembling, hair on the neck becoming erect. Sadness can be seen to range from *distress* (upset, sad, tearful, or crying) to *anguish* (suffering, tortured, or tormented). We would see a raised inner portion of eyebrows, a lowering of mouth corners, and crying or sobbing. Figure 8 shows the facial expressions in column one, the emotions in column two, and the affects in column three.

Four of these six facial expressions are our primary emotions of anger, fear, sadness, and joy; the other two are shock and disgust. All play a crucial part in human sexuality. It is a vital link in human connectedness and emotionality that we can instantaneously feel an emotion, a reaction, in response to another and can trigger the same in others, too. We are recognising and comprehending all these non-verbal communications. In the 1990s, Ekman expanded this list to include some more complex emotions, such as contempt, embarrass-

Surprise	Shock, may trigger the fight or flight response, or freeze, like a rabbit in headlights	brows arch eyes open wide to expose more white jaw drops slightly
Anger	Tells us something is not OK, we need to take action – Fight	brows lowered lips pressed firmly eyes bulging
Fear	Tells us something is not OK, we need to withdraw – Flight	brows raised eyes open mouth opens slightly
Sadness	Sorrow, our experience of grief, sadness, loss, separation distress – Panic	lowering of mouth corners raise inner portion of brows
Happiness	Joy, things are OK	raising and lowering of mouth corners
Disgust	A socially learnt concept of repulsion, rejection and shame	upper lip is raised nose bridge is wrinkled cheeks raised

Figure 8. Six human facial expressions.

ment, guilt, shame, and the more positive feelings of amusement, contentment, pride in achievement, relief, sensory pleasure, and satisfaction.

Exercise   Emotional awareness 2

Think about your awareness of and reactions to other people's emotions. Can you identify the facial expressions, body postures, tone and pitch of voice in others that alert you to which emotions they are expressing? Think about the primary emotions of anger, fear, sadness and joy; and then also other expressions of emotion like disappointment or confusion. Consider the following:

When I see someone else crying, I feel . . .
and I think. . .

When I see someone else looking frightened, I feel . . .
and I think . . .

When I see someone else being angry, I feel . . .
and I think. . . .

When I see someone else being happy, I feel . . .
and I think . . .

Notice which of these emotions in others that you find it easier or more difficult to respond or relate to. How does this relate to how you experience your own emotions; is there a similar pattern, or are you able to tolerate expressions in others that you don't allow for yourself? Again, how does this mirror your childhood experiences?

Reflect on what you have written and identify one thing you would like to change and consider how you could do that.

Seven human imperatives

Invaluable work has been done by Panksepp (1998) and Sunderland (2007) in integrating knowledge from neuroscience with psychotherapeutic understanding. Building on their work, we can review our understanding of human sexuality by looking beyond the sexual drive as a reproductive urge. Panksepp identifies some brain circuits that will trigger predictable behaviours when certain areas of the brain are stimulated. Those he calls the seeker, lust, caring, and joy, all induce feel-good chemistry such as dopamine, endorphins, oxytocin, and prolactin and activate the basal forebrain. The others distress us and our limbic system.

- *Seeker*: Ecstasy, happiness exploration.
- *Lust*: Consummatory behaviour, hunger, and the procreative urge.
- *Care*: Love, nurturing, and social bonding.
- *Joy*: The need for touch, to rough and tumble play.
- *Rage*: Anger, frustration, thwarted drive.
- *Fear*: Terror, fear, anxiety.
- *Panic*: Utter misery, grief, loss. Separation anxiety, abandonment.

Recent studies in neuroscience have taught us a lot about human functioning. Most research regarding sexuality has been derived from studying animal reproductive patterns, which are then applied to humans, resulting in a focus on the reproductive model of sex. We can, however, explore this in a wider sense when we include other reasons for humans being sexual. By reviewing current research with a new paradigm we can consider the socialising and relational issues involved in sexual attraction and sexual functioning. If we remove lust, as the reproductive imperative, from the equation for the moment, we can consider what role the others might play in human sexuality and our sexual appetites. We could see fight (rage), flight (fear), and panic as survival reactions that move us *away from* or against others, and caring, curiosity (seeker), and joy as drives with a socialising function; which move us *towards* others (Figure 9).

Rage and fear are the fight and flight responses, both of which activate the amygdala and hippocampus in the limbic system, quickly triggering the release of adrenalin for urgent action, and, more slowly, cortisol for stamina. These hormones disrupt links to the frontal lobes, impairing our thinking. We need to be able to get on with it, not think about how we feel. The fight response can be experienced mildly, as irritation, through to rage, when levels are high. Fear can be mild or

SURVIVAL	Reactions against other
Fight	danger, need to take action
Flight	need to get away, withdraw
Panic	abandonment, loss, separation distress

Figure 9.   The survival brain circuits.

be terrifying; we might be able to withdraw or become frozen, like a rabbit in headlights. Disassociation and out of body experiences might be triggered. Panic activates the hypothalamus, which triggers a sudden drop in oxytocin, the bonding hormone. Panksepp identifies panic as a state of separation anxiety due to loss of attachment. This is an important differentiation, as we often relate to panic as anxiety, as a fear emotion. Reframing this experience in connection to attachment, as a relational experience, could alter our thinking and treatment strategies for panic attacks.

The relational, socialising drives are vital for us as humans (Figure 10). Our caring circuit moderates our empathy skills, our desires to nurture and soothe that are crucial to our survival. Because our infants and children are so physically and emotionally dependent on adults to stay alive, let alone thrive, we humans need more than a good live birth rate to maintain our species; our young need to be kept alive. Empathy is a vital human attribute for a healthy society; it is important that we can and do feel compassion for others, so we can help the more vulnerable and ensure survival. The issue of empathy and the opposites, lack of compassion and objectification, are important issues of our day and our social structure, specifically so in the arena of sexuality. A lack of empathy allows humans to hurt others without regard to how it might feel, without care.

Our incessant inquisitiveness as humans might seem to get us into trouble at times, but we probably would not do much without it. It is our curiosity circuit that encourages the infant to reach out, or motivates the desire to move, first to crawl, and later, to walk. As children, our curiosity is rampant and can be a source of exasperation to many parents, teachers, carers, and siblings, who often do not know the

SOCIALISING	Move us towards other
Caring	our capacity to have empathy and look after other people
Curiosity	our interest in others and the world around us
Play and physical contact	our need for touch and fun with others

Figure 10.   The socialising brain circuits.

answers to the why, how, and what questions of our youngsters. It is our curiosity, motivated by the brain chemical dopamine, that gets us to explore and to consider "what if". Many things we use in our modern world were invented because of someone's curiosity, and their imagination. Someone thought what if we could move around in a vehicle, or fly through the sky, or have a device like a mobile phone?

An urge for play and touch has been identified in the young of many mammals and is probably central to human sexual urges, too. Infants explore their environment first through their senses: sight, sound, taste, smell, and touch. Anything felt in their hands will primarily be moved to the mouth to be tasted and smelled. Physical contact is of vital importance to children, who often seek touch and physical connection with their carers. Research on children in orphanages showed that, despite being fed and clothed (their physical needs cared for), a lack of touch, of physical contact with carers in the first few years of life had led to brain damage (Chugani et al., 2001). Frontal lobes (necessary for thinking and choosing) had not grown sufficiently and neural pathways linking to the limbic system were not developed either. Such damage has also been seen in brain scans of children in Britain whose emotional needs have not been met (Batmanghelidjh, 2007).

Exercise   Towards and away

Think about some recent incidents where you definitely felt attracted towards someone or something that was happening, or where you felt repelled. Choose one of each and consider each in more depth to identify details about why you were attracted or not.

Now think about yourself sexually. What types of experiences and encounters with others attract you (turn you on) and what repels you (turn you off)? Think about this with regard to your physical body and sensations, your emotions and feelings, and your belief system and preferences.

Reflect on what you have written and consider if there are things you would like to change, and, if so, how you could do so.

Us and them

Building on the work of his father, John Bowlby (1988), Richard Bowlby (2004) has shown that although children seek "rough and tumble" play with others, the quality of this contact is vital. A primary attachment figure is often the mother, but not necessarily so; it is the main carer, the person who most often attends the child's calls of physical and emotional distress. When this is experienced as secure, consistent, and reliable, the child is soothed by the interventions of the adult, gradually learning to self-soothe and develop an inner sense of the world as a safe place. When soothing is not offered, the rage, fear, and panic circuits become more activated and more entrenched. This hyper-arousal, together with damage to frontal lobes, can be disastrous for a growing child, causing long-term difficulties with self-esteem and relationships as adults.

Richard Bowlby's work, a twenty-one year study on attachment, showed the equal importance of a secondary attachment figure, usually, but not necessarily, the father. This person would be more likely to engage in rough and tumble play with the child, which can develop its sense of confidence in the outside world, of being in the public realm. However, he found that bullying or a critical attitude from this adult role would produce the opposite: a lack of public confidence, again bringing problems for adults' social or work lives. Humans are constantly responding to their outside environment with self-preserving, hardwired brain reflexes. We are also social beings, interested in, and seeking out, others to interact with. These socialising drives are modulated mainly around pleasure or pain, which can be either physical or emotional, usually both. Pain and pleasure are both experienced in an area known as the PAG, which connects with the hippocampus in the limbic system. Neurochemicals, such as dopamine and serotonin, are seen as part of a "reward or punishment" system. Essentially, when our encounters result in pleasure, we continue, we move towards that which is giving us pleasure. When they result in pain, one of the survival modes of fight, flight, or panic will come into play as we react against the pain and move away.

So, what about sex and sexuality? The three socialising drives of caring, curiosity, and play and physical touch seem very pertinent to how and why humans express their sexuality and the sexual behaviours they display. Sexual behaviours could be seen as a playground where adults get their "rough and tumble" play; how much rough and how much play is surely a question for consideration, given Bowlby's findings. If the fight or flight circuits are activated, the system is flooded with adrenalin, possibly alongside the pleasure chemicals serotonin and dopamine. Can our fundamental ability to distinguish pain (i.e., move away from) and pleasure (move towards) become confused?

Our curiosity circuit is clearly triggered in sexual attraction, sexual desire, and sexual arousal. We become interested and intrigued; we want to know more, see more, and feel more. We often want to care for, protect, and tend to our lovers, maybe to cook for them, take them out, bring pleasure, and make them happy. These aspects speak much more to the relationship and intimacy needs of our sexuality than the biology of reproduction that tends to be focused on. It implies some much wider needs than a sexual act.

Exercise   Conscious breathing

Take yourself to your safe space when you have at least thirty minutes in which you will not be disturbed. Get yourself into a comfortable sitting position, close your eyes, and allow a few minutes to settle and begin to relax. Notice sounds around you and thoughts you have, and let them go.

Focus on your breathing, just noticing, not judging. Scan down your body and imagine any tensions leaving with the out-breath; allow yourself to slowly relax. Feel the rhythmic pattern of your breath coming in and leaving, just noticing and being aware of your body. If you become distracted, don't worry; just take your attention back to your breathing.

Place one hand on your heart and one hand on your genitals and continue to focus on your out-breath then your in-breath. Just sit for a few minutes to get a sense of a connection between these two parts of your body.

With your eyes closed, think about someone or something that attracts you sexually. Use your imagination to allow allow a sexual charge to build and see if and how your breathing changes.

Then make a choice to change what you are thinking about so as to reduce your arousal. Notice any changes to your breathing pattern. Experiment with using your breath to increase and then decrease your arousal. Notice, as well, what thoughts and imaginings help with doing this.

Reflect on this exercise afterwards and write about any thoughts or feelings you have.

Sexual arousal in humans often triggers a desire for an other, to reach out and touch, both literally and metaphorically, to make contact, connection. Our circuits of curiosity, care, and joy are activated, and move us towards socialisation. They trigger feel-good hormones, the reward system of the body. Touching skin and being touched and held, cuddled, releases oxytocin, the love and bonding hormone. Oxytocin, which floods the body during sexual arousal and peaks at orgasm, is seen as an evolutionary mutation of vasopressin, which triggers reproductive behaviour in mammals (Panksepp, 1998).

Getting hot

Sexual desire can refer to a more abstract concept of our sexual drive or libido, where we might think about the strength or intensity of our desire. For the purpose of understanding, we are separating the impact of sexual desire on the mind, body, brain, and emotions. In reality, all aspects cause reactions in, and response to, the others.

When we are "turned on", sexual energy is set in motion, triggering actions and reactions. Sexual desire is controlled and affected by hormones and brain chemicals. It is affected by physical stimuli, such as sight, sound, touch, taste, and smell, and also psychological stimuli, such as imagination and mood, as well as social and cultural factors. Sexual desire can trigger a yearning and longing for contact with an other, especially to touch and be touched and an oral desire to kiss and be kissed. It can trigger physical sexual arousal, but not necessarily. Many feelings can be generated, including excitement and curiosity, anticipation and hope. There is often happiness and euphoria, feelings of wellbeing. There can also be the grief, fear, and anger of frustrations and disappointments.

We can distinguish sexual desire, the activation of neurochemicals from the brain, from sexual arousal, the physiological impacts on the body. Brain activation will also include reactions from the memory centres. Desire also activates our minds and our imagination, which feeds our arousal with sexual fantasy and anticipation of pleasure. Just imagining can turn us on. It will include input from our belief systems, preferences, and choices. We can also become sexually aroused through physical stimulation. Physical arousal includes a heightened arousal of all our senses and the nervous system, which also can lead to an agitation and disruption to body systems such as sleep and eating patterns. It affects our breathing and heart rate, and our temperature rises; vaginal lubrication is released from the bartholins glands in women and other erogenous zones are awakened.

When we are turned on, there is tension in the motor muscles of the body, but relaxation of the smooth muscle in the genitals, which, together with an increase of blood flow to the pelvic area, facilitates erection. Generally, sexual activity is good for the body, regulating hormones, invigorating the circulatory and respiratory systems, and toning organs, glands, and muscles. It helps to protect against the many conditions and illnesses caused by the disregulation of any of the above (Figure 11).

Brain The back brain, the limbic system, fight and flight reflexes, urges, desire, memories and history ■ Neurochemicals – Dopamine, Vasopressin, Serotonin, PEA ■ Activation of memory centres flashbacks to previous sexual arousals/traumas	Mind The frontal lobes. Thinking, choices and imagination. Beliefs and values ■ Imagination – potentials and possibilities ■ Preoccupation about choices and actions – ways to make it happen ■ Social and cultural beliefs – promotion and prohibitions
Sexual arousal	
Body The physical body. Sight, sound, taste, smell, touching, being touched. Sensual and sexual arousal ■ Increase in heartbeat, body temperature and breathing ■ Tightness in stomach ■ Stirring in genitals ■ Heightened arousal of senses and nervous system ■ Agitation and disruption to body systems – food, sleep	Emotion Feelings and emotions. Love, loss, fear, anger. Energy in motion ■ Yearning and longing for contact with other – to kiss, to touch ■ Excitement and curiosity ■ Anticipation and hope ■ Happiness, euphoria – feelings of wellbeing ■ Frustrations and disappointments Fight, flight, panic, shame, shock

Figure 11. The impact of desire.

Exercise   Sexual touch

Make a time for yourself in your safe space. Make it warm.

Take your clothes off or just those covering your genitals, sit for a few moments and settle. Close your eyes and put your hands on your genitals. Spend a few minutes just breathing and noticing how you are feeling and what you are thinking.

At first, keep your eyes closed and gently touch and explore your penis or vulva with your fingers. Explore touching the outer and the inner vulva lips and inside the vagina, or the penis, including the foreskin (if you have one), the scrotum, and the anus.

Explore the rest of your body, touching your skin all over. Notice where it feels sensuous and where it feels erotic. Experiment with touching your skin with your hands and fingers, also through clothing or other materials.

As you touch yourself, notice any sensations in your body and any feelings evoked. Notice what it feels like to touch yourself (the sensation to your fingers) and also what it feels like being touched (the sensations in your genitals).

Open your eyes or keep them closed while you experiment with your touch, paying attention to what you like, what feels good, and also what you don't like. Play with touching yourself more firmly and more gently, making your touch faster or slower.

Notice what touch you like and consciously continue to touch, to pleasure yourself. Experiment with your breathing, deeper or shorter breaths, to see which increase or reduce your pleasure. Notice what ideas, desires, thoughts, and imaginations are triggered while you are doing this.

For this exercise, you are invited to stop once your arousal is high, not to continue to orgasm, but to just sit and breathe and experience yourself in high arousal and be conscious about that. Notice what you feel in your body and what you are thinking about. Allow time for your arousal to subside as you no longer feed the charge. How easy or difficult is it for you to stop, and just be conscious of what is happening?

Take some time to reflect on and write about what you have experienced.

Build the charge

Once a sexual charge has been triggered, it proceeds through various stages, as explained in Figure 12. This is based on the Masters and Johnson model (1966, 2004) but expanded to show the distinction between orgasm and ejaculation. All of the elements of sensuality, feelings, and emotions will be building this charge. Any breaks to arousal, that is any "turn-offs", can stop the charge from continuing. And equally, any "turn-ons" can be used to restore the charge and bring it back on line. This is a generalised model and you might wish to refer back to exercises on self-pleasuring to consider how your pattern of arousal may be similar or different.

1. Non-aroused is how we are before a stimulus triggers an arousal.
2. Excitement can last from a few minutes to several hours:
    - we become "turned on" and begin to build a charge of sexual energy;
    - muscle tension increases;
    - heart rate quickens and breathing is accelerated;
    - skin may become flushed;
    - nipples become hardened or erect;

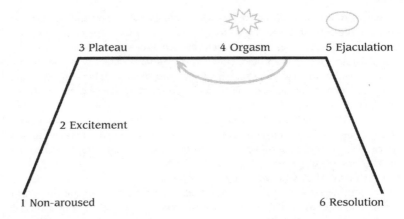

Figure 12.   Six stages of sexual arousal.

- smooth muscle in the clitoris and penis relax, allowing erection;
- blood flow to the genitals increases, resulting in further erection of the clitoris or penis;
- vaginal lubrication begins;
- the woman's breasts become fuller and the vaginal walls begin to swell;
- the man's testicles swell, his scrotum tightens, and he begins secreting a lubricating liquid—pre-ejaculate.

3.   Plateau extends to the brink of orgasm:
- relaxing, letting go to enjoying a heightened state of sexual arousal;
- the changes begun in the excitement phase are intensified;
- the vagina continues to swell from increased blood flow, and the vaginal walls turn a dark purple;
- the woman's clitoris becomes highly sensitive and the glans retracts under the clitoral hood to avoid direct stimulation;
- the man's testicles are withdrawn up into the scrotum;
- breathing, heart rate, and blood pressure continue to increase;
- muscle spasms may begin in the feet, face, and hands;
- muscle tension increases.

4.   Orgasm is the shortest of the phases:
- blood pressure, heart rate, and breathing are at their highest rates, with a rapid intake of oxygen;
- a rash or "sex flush" might appear over the entire body;

- involuntary muscle contractions begin, particularly in the pelvic floor;
- the muscles of the vagina and base of the penis, the uterus, and prostate gland undergo rhythmic contractions;
- surges of hormones and neurochemicals trigger a reflex action through the nervous system and the release of sexual tension throughout the whole body;
- after orgasm the body returns to its pre-orgasmic phase, and can experience multiple orgasms.

5. Ejaculation can happen at the same time as orgasm or separately:
    - rhythmic contractions of the pelvic floor muscles result in the release of ejaculatory fluid from the prostate and seminal glands in men, and from the paraurethral glands in women;
    - after ejaculation, the body returns to stage 1; non-aroused and needs a recovery time before it can become aroused again.

6. Resolution:
    - during resolution, the body slowly returns to its normal level of functioning, and swollen and erect body parts return to their previous size and colour;
    - the duration of the refractory period varies and usually lengthens with advancing age.
    - this phase is marked by a general sense of wellbeing, enhanced intimacy, and, often, fatigue.

Understanding the stages of arousal can be useful to clarify any difficulties we might be having. First, we need to distinguish between desire (do we *want* to be sexual?) and arousal (are we *able* to respond physically?). If our attempt to be sexual is matching our desire but we are having difficulty with physiological arousal, knowing at what stage of the arousal process this is happening can give us clues about how to encourage our body to respond. For example, if excitement is not building at all, or increasing but then stopping, we might want to slow down and focus on what does build our sexual charge. Learning that our sexual charge can ebb and flow is useful; knowing that if we lose an erection it does not necessarily mean it is all over, depending on our choices and attitudes.

The plateau stage is an important awareness in psychosexual health. We seem to believe the charge builds and builds until release, so when we reach plateau it might be experienced as a decline. Often, at this point, we become more aware of our thoughts and feelings, as well as our sensory experiences, which can feel disconcerting as we seem to believe we are supposed to be lost in it all. This also requires a consciousness about being sexual, and, therefore, a relative ease about being so. Sexual shame can get in the way of sexual self-esteem and will be discussed later.

Separating orgasm and ejaculation as differing stages allows us to think about our sexual behaviours in a new way also. Ejaculation, obviously correlated with our "reproductive model of sex" thinking, brings the physiological process of sexual arousal to a conclusion, albeit temporarily. Orgasm, however, takes the process back to the pre-orgasmic stage, allowing for the possibility of multiple orgasms.

For women, however, the distinctions between arousal and desire are more complex. It is known that both penile erection and vaginal lubrication can also occur in response to unwanted touch, for example during sexual abuse. This can confuse people, who believe there must have been some desire present. Such physiological responses are reflexes triggered through the autonomic nervous system purely by touch, which indicates we need to consider not just the ability to be aroused, but the subjective experience of that: what a person feels about what is happening in their body. Seeing that many women did not seem to conform to the linear model of arousal described above, Whipple and Brash-McGreer (1997) proposed a circular sexual response pattern (Figure 13). They suggest that pleasant and satisfying sexual experiences might have a reinforcing effect on a woman,

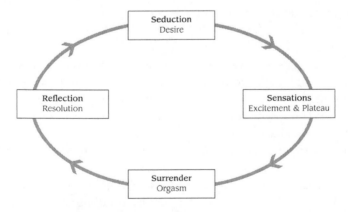

Figure 13.   A circular sexual response pattern.

leading to the seduction phase of the next sexual experience. If, during reflection, the sexual experience did not provide pleasure and satisfaction, the woman might not have a desire to repeat the experience.

Following from this, Basson (2001) constructed a new model of female sexual response, which acknowledges the importance of emotional intimacy, sexual stimuli, and relationship satisfaction in female sexual response (Figure 14). She believes that although women may experience spontaneous sexual desire and interest in some circumstances, many women, especially those in long-term relationships, are more likely to participate in sexual activity in response to a partner or through a desire for intimacy. She identifies a need for "willingness", which she calls "seeking out or being receptive to" a sexual encounter. Once aroused, her desire will then emerge and motivate her to continue. Basson argues that the motivations for sexual activity for women is not necessarily the goal of orgasm, but, rather, personal satisfaction, which can manifest as the physical satisfaction of orgasm and/or the emotional satisfaction of feeling intimacy and connection with a partner.

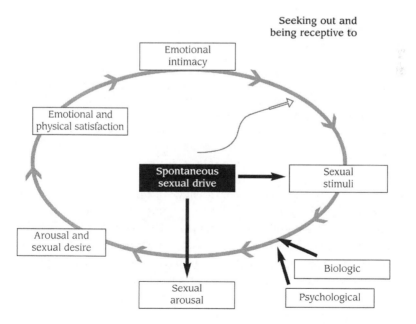

Figure 14. Basson's model of female sexual response.

This model is particularly useful for women during the menopause and for men during the aging process. In later life, we are not so driven sexually by our hormones and need to find a new way into our desire than how we have been used to. Northrup (1995, 2003) explains how rather than becoming "hormone deficient" at menopause, the amount of oestrogen now needed in a woman's body is changing as she no longer needs such levels for ovulation. In fact, her whole endocrine system is transitioning, so that, in time, her adrenal system will change androgens into oestrogen to provide the levels she now needs. The most important care during the peri-menopause years, while this change is happening, is of the adrenal system, to reduce the stresses which overactivate it. Discovering more about the specific ways we feel turned on, emotionally and physically, can help this process. Rather than feeling a lack of desire, many discover that the gateway to their desire has changed. Allowing for this and exploring new avenues into sexual activities often results in a renewed interest and fulfilling experiences of sex. Another excellent resource book for women is *Becoming Orgasmic* (Heinman & LoPiccolo (1998).

Exercise   Sexual fantasy

Take some time to think about what you have learnt about yourself physically and emotionally with regard to your sexuality. Write a sexual fantasy in as much detail as you want. Imagine a scenario where you are receiving exactly what you want: for example, where you are and who with, what happens, in what order.

When you have done this, compare your fantasy with your real-life experiences. Is this particular fantasy one you prefer to keep in the world of your imagination, or would you like to share it, or part of it, with a partner?

All together now

We have explored our mind, our beliefs and thinking, and the physiology of our body and our brain during sexual arousal. Let us consider now linking it all back together. The brain releases chemicals which trigger changes in the body, setting energy in motion, triggering thoughts, memories, triggering more chemicals, and so on: a chain of events, a cycle of interaction. This cycle can also be seen as a circuit; it can be switched on and it can be switched off.

A trigger to arousal can start in any section, but will activate the others (Figure 15). It might start from an external sensory stimulus,

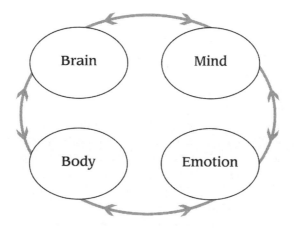

Figure 15. A circuit of arousal.

such as sight or touch, or an internal stimulus, such as a thought or a memory. Once triggered, it causes an autonomic reaction in the body to arousal. We can turn off this arousal and cut the circuit if, for example, our thinking tells us it is not appropriate right now, or we do not want to follow the urge right now. It is important as humans that we are not slaves to our drives and can exercise some choices. As said before, we are constantly negotiating with our drives and urges. We may suppress, switch off, the desire to laugh, to shout, or cry. We may feel a hunger that we put off until we can eat next. We can do the same sexually. Our body–brain–mind is always in dialogue.

If we feel sexual desire and sexual arousal in our body we can choose to switch it off, which will break the circuit and stop further production of neurochemicals, which are triggering the physical changes; physical arousal will then subside. We cannot change how we feel, or what our reactions are, but we can choose how we respond: whether we "allow" a continuation of excitation to build through the stages of arousal, or whether we break the circuit. Knowing in greater detail what breaks the circuit and what enhances our arousal can help us to switch it back on if we want to.

Sometimes, this switch-off can happen more unconsciously. For example, if we are attempting to "perform" but do not really want to be in the scenario we are in, with the person we are with, or doing what we are doing, our body, our physiological arousal, can be halted. Similarly, if our feelings or values are not in synchronisation with our actions, our circuit of arousal can be broken. Again, understanding where in the circuit we are experiencing the rupture can help us to re-evaluate our behaviour and either repair the break or choose not to continue.

We rarely take time to contemplate all the different components to human behaviour, mainly because the communication between our brain reactions, our body sensations, our emotions, and our thoughts, all happen so quickly. The actions that we take, how we behave, is the consequence of myriad issues we have addressed so far. Our history, our beliefs, and our body responses will all have an input into the decision making which precedes action. It is important to acknowledge our capabilities and choices in relationship to our sexual urges and arousal. The model that we are mostly likely to see (on television, for example), usually implies we have little control: that once we are turned on, we will be taken over until we have fulfilled that urge by the physical act of sex. This is obviously not true; how much responsibility we take for ourselves sexually is a matter for this book.

Exercise   Sexual stimulation

Make a time for yourself in your safe space. Make it warm. This exercise is similar to that of sexual touch, but develops in a different way.

Take your clothes off or just those covering your genitals, sit for a few moments and settle. Close your eyes and put your hands on your genitals. Spend a few minutes just breathing and noticing how you are feeling and what you are thinking.

At first, keep your eyes closed and gently touch and explore your penis or vulva with your fingers. Explore touching the outer and the inner vulva lips and inside the vagina, or the penis, including the foreskin (if you have one), the scrotum, and the anus. Explore and play more with the other parts of your body that also create an erotic charge.

As you touch yourself, notice any sensations in your body and any feelings evoked. Notice what it feels like to touch yourself (the sensation to your fingers) and also what it feels like being touched (the sensations in your genitals).

Open your eyes or keep them closed while you experiment with your touch, paying attention to what you like, what feels good, and also what you don't like. Play with touching yourself more firmly and more gently, making your touch faster or slower. Play with touching and then stopping and just holding yourself and breathing, and then touching again.

Notice what touch you like and consciously continue to touch, to pleasure yourself. Experiment with your breathing, deeper or shorter breaths, to see which increase or reduce your pleasure. Notice what ideas, desires, thoughts, and imaginations are triggered while you are doing this.

For this exercise, you are invited to continue your pleasuring to orgasm, and to remain mindful and conscious of what you are feeling in your body. Notice any thoughts that might arise. Notice your imagination; how are you feeding your desire?

Take some time to reflect on and write about what you have experienced. How easy was it for you to stay connected to what was happening in your body? How do you feel having done this and what do you think about it?

Go with the flow

Sexual arousal starts an energy charge that passes through the circuit as described above. If all aspects are in tune, it will continue the circuit and build the charge up through the stages of arousal of excitation and up to the plateau. Given the right factors, it is a natural reflex to orgasm and/or ejaculate in response to sexual arousal.

Each of the aspects of mind, brain, body, and emotion is affected by sexual arousal and each has needs, too. Our sexual arousal circuit will flow at its easiest when these needs are met. We will be affected internally and also by our outside environment: where we are and whom we are with. If our sexual activities and behaviour are acceptable to our thinking, memories, and beliefs, then feel-good chemicals will flow; if not, we might produce adrenalin, which could trigger fight or flight emotions and/or shut down physical arousal.

There can also be extraordinary and unusual responses to and during sexual arousal when considering a history of sexual violence. Owing to the impacts on the limbic system, there can be unwanted arousal to stimuli evocative of events. There can be confusing beliefs about, and responses to, the distinctions between pain and pleasure, what is in our best interest and what is not. Survival strategies can take over, triggering fear or rage and perhaps freeze or disassociation.

Imagination and fantasy are really important in sexuality, too. Just imagining can turn us on. When our sensuality is being turned on, and not off, and we are receiving the quality and quantity of touch and, specifically, genital stimulation that we enjoy; then orgasm/ejaculation will be reflexive responses. Unwelcome thoughts, feelings, or emotions can also switch off the circuit, as can stress or illness; these issues will be addressed in more detail later.

The best environment to enhance our sexual pleasure is when all aspects of our body–mind–brain–emotions are being satisfied. Primarily, sexuality is a relationship with yourself. When we know what turns us on, sensually and sexually, what satisfies our beliefs and choices, what harmonises our emotions, then we allow the sexual charge to flow, enjoy the pleasures of a sexual experience, and are satiated through orgasmic release. The bio-neurochemical experience of sexual activity is great for us: body, heart, and soul.

Given the pain and struggles of human life, it is a wonderful gift to be able to experience sexual pleasure and physical satiation, with all its benefits. It can be blissful also, emotionally and existentially, to be able to connect with and be intimate with another, to play and share making love together. Sexual expression can take many forms, including dancing, masturbating, or being sexual with someone else. How we express our sexuality and how we relate to others are influenced by all the things we have been discussing.

Drawing together all the issues and factors we have identified, we can see our drive towards being sexual includes the pleasure principle and the erotic principle. It is also our fire energy, about creativity, and fuels our passions, including love and spirituality. Given our reactivity and our ability to reflect and choose, to some extent, how we will react, how do we want to behave sexually? Drawing together our sexual beliefs and preferences, our physical desire, brain and body, how do we want to meet and be sexual with another?

Exploring the feelings and emotions evoked by our sexual energy charge, neurochemistry and body changes, is the next strand of our story. Having an in-depth understanding of our sexual physiology is a bit like understanding how our digestive system works: we do not need to know in order to be able to enjoy eating. (It is interesting how little we know about sexual, as opposed to reproductive, functioning.) Equally, people do not need to be told about how to have sex. This book is a more a manual about sexual nutrition; what our body does, why it does it, and with what consequences. We know innately how to be sexual; we are exploring why we think, respond, and act as we do. So, let us move on to emotion and feelings.

Exercise   Review of Part III

Read back through the exercises for this section and what you have written in your journal. Take some time to reflect on your exploration and to evaluate your work. Which exercises did you like and which ones did you not like? Think about why.

What have you discovered about your instinctual drives? What have you discovered about your emotional intelligence, and what upsets you in relationships and what makes you feel good?

What have you discovered about your desire in terms of what you think, how you like to be touched, and what fires your imagination?

Is there anything you want to change? If so, how could you do that?

Are there any exercises that you would like to do again? If so, notice what is similar or different if you do them a second time.

Talk to someone, write or draw something about how you are thinking and feeling having worked on this section.

PART IV

EMOTION: FEELINGS AND INTUITION

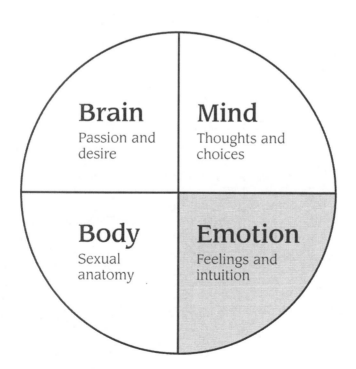

Emotion, body, brain, and mind.

Emotion

Dark side of the moon

In this section, we shall discuss the range of emotions and feelings that we might have about the facets of sexuality that have been introduced so far. We shall also begin to draw these elements together, to consider how they interact and to further develop an integrative model for sexuality. In Part I, "Mind: thoughts and choices", many areas were introduced to explore our current social and cultural beliefs and values about sexuality. These included our use of language, our attitudes to sexuality and to pleasure, and concepts such as the "reproductive" model of sex. We discussed options and choices for a healthy sexual diet and sexual self-esteem. We will revisit some of these issues having learnt in more detail about how our bodies and our brain work with regard to sexuality.

Part II described our sexual anatomy in detail, not just the genitals, but also other vital body systems, such as the endocrine and nervous systems. It also explained the various stages of the sexual arousal process and outlined our physiological sexual potential. Part III described the neurochemistry of sexual arousal and the role of the brain in sexuality and sexual functioning. By reframing neuroscientific information about brain circuits, we can gain a deeper understanding of human sexuality, seeing our sex urge as much more than a vital human imperative to reproduce.

The "socialising" brain circuits of caring, curiosity, play, and touch can clearly be seen to be relevant to our sexuality. We will explore our feelings about these aspects, rarely discussed and not taught in schools. We can consider if these topics were central to our thinking and cultural values, and whether this would affect our sexual attitudes and behaviours. The "reactive" circuits of fight, flight, or panic certainly pertain to sexuality and affairs of the heart through anger, fear, or loss of a loved one. These emotions receive a bad press as the "negative" emotions. We do not like to feel "bad", and, thus, culturally hide these feelings. This hiding creates a shadow, a dark side, and sexuality certainly has a dark side in our culture—sexual violence. To contemplate a model of psychosexual *health*, we must be willing to look into this corner of our culture and give it a good shake, blow out the cobwebs, and see what is there.

Information about sex and sexuality has definitely increased in the past decade and our attitudes have, no doubt, changed also. It would be useful to evaluate the impact of this liberalisation on our sexual self-esteem. It does seem that many topics related to sexuality still raise plenty of feelings for most people and generate feelings of shame. We do not yet have a cultural ease about sex or sexuality. We have far too many sexual crimes, and too high rates of sexual addiction and sexually transmitted infections. After exploring these issues, we shall focus on creating a homeodynamic model for sexual self-esteem.

Exercise   Your dark side

Write about how you feel good about yourself sexually and how you don't feel good. Explore in depth what you don't feel good about. Is it your beliefs, your body, your behaviours, or your experiences?

When you have done this, reflect on what you have written and consider the context for your words in terms of your upbringing. How have your beliefs and experiences been influenced by what you were taught, or learnt, as a child or young person?

Truth and lies

It can feel difficult to imagine sexual self-esteem for us as individuals and as a culture. We are exploring some areas that seem to be specifically uncomfortable for us. A reproductive model of sex is so entrenched in our thinking that we hardly notice how our language and concepts revolve around it. Our very varied experiences of being sexual become channelled into a limited notion of sex as an act, most often, of heterosexual intercourse and other expressions become marginalised. We are discouraged from talking about sexuality and from valuing our emotional and relational needs. We seem to believe we are only reactive sexually; we are not encouraged to be reflective and make conscious choices about our sexual lives.

It can be difficult to develop a sense of sexual self-esteem when we do not have a cultural sex-positive attitude. Children pick up our embarrassment about using even basic language about their bodies. Parents and relatives delight in an infant's discovery of their toes and fingers but not of their genitals, which can trigger responses from embarrassment to anger. This is probably our first sexually shaming experience.

I recently witnessed a scene where a two-year-old was asking her mother a question about her genitals in front of me, another mother, and two slightly older girls. After much giggling, the embarrassed mother referred to her daughter's vulva as "your not-a-willy", much to the children's bemusement. Shere Hite (1994) raised the question of what impact it must have on girls' experience of themselves sexually when they can see that they have external organs but they are not named and often ignored. When toddlers ask about the differences between boys and girls that they can see, they are often answered with descriptions of penises (outside the body) and vaginas (inside the body) and, in time, told about males and females "making babies" through intercourse. That females have a clitoris is not mentioned much; if it is, it is often misrepresented in size and function. Women's external genitalia, the vulva, is rarely referred to. Even in contemporary sex education aimed at teenagers, the word "vagina" is confusingly used to describe both the vulva and the vagina itself (Boynton, 2011).

The adult world of sexuality must seem so confusing to our children; there are so many mixed messages, with sex being used to sell many things, but, at the same time, much embarrassment can be generated in adults when we talk about sexual matters. Sex is everywhere around, so obviously very important to adults, yet which bits and why must be hard to fathom. Our fixation with sexualised breasts is obvious, yet women are expected to be discreet, if not hidden, when breastfeeding an infant. More attention is paid to being thin, rather than feeling good about having a healthy body mass index (the ratio between our weight, height, and body frame).

When teenagers begin to experience their emerging sexuality, hormonal and physiological changes are generating plenty of feelings and emotions as well. Yet, our focus seems to be on looking sexy rather than feeling sexy, and that being sexual is about having intercourse with someone, rather than an aspect of growing up that is raising very many thoughts, feelings, and questions. As they do not generally have free conversation and get to explore these issues with their parents, carers, or other adults around, young people rely on their peer group and, more recently, by accessing pornography on the Internet (Richardson, 2009). This promotes an objectifying, non-relational approach, portraying sexual acts rather than any emotions or intimacy. We will talk about love later.

Starting with ourselves, within a homeodynamic model, we can more consciously create the sort of sexual life we want. We understand our brain reactions and our body's sexual potential. We can use our emotions as basic information, as an immediate response about whether or not we like what is happening. By becoming explicit about our thinking (our beliefs and values), we can create a framework to further inform how we might want to act and how we want to behave sexually.

Exercise   Your truths

Write two lists, one about the things you think are true and one about the things you think are lies about what you see and hear about sexuality, in the media or from family, friends, or peers.

Of the things you think are lies, consider why such things might be said and believed by others. Clarify for yourself your list of truths; add any more that you think are missed by us culturally and think out for yourself why you think they are truths.

Full of feelings

We use the word "feelings" to mean many things, such as an emotion, a sensation, a thought, or a hunch. It can be useful to separate them within the homeodynamic model for health. Talking about "feeling sexual", for example, can mean several things. Having a feeling and choosing whether or not to act on it, is a central tenet of this book. Figure 16 shows a homeodynamic model of feelings.

Whenever a reaction is triggered in us, our neurochemistry responds, causing physiological effects, activating energy moving through the body, generating thoughts about all this, and immediately more reactions, responses, and so on. We are exploring a complex, interweaved web of "being human". Understanding these aspects of our "feelings" can be helpful to simplify the different strands and provide problem-solving tools.

This is specifically so in relationship to sexuality. To separate "feeling sexual" into components of a physical urge, or an emotional desire or a thought, can inform us in more detail about what we really want. One strand might mean we feel turned on and want to be sexual, with ourselves or with another; another might mean we want some emotional closeness or intimacy, or we might want both. Such distinctions can help guide us to getting our deeper needs met.

In the "Mind" section of this book, we have explored our thinking, beliefs, and values, and how these have an impact on our experience of our sexuality and, therefore, our sexual behaviour. In the "Body"

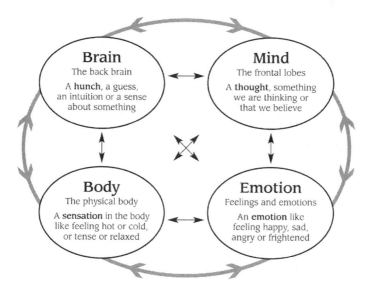

Figure 16. A homeodynamic model of feelings.

section, our biological capacities were described, and the physical sensations of feeling sexual. The "Brain" section described the neuro-chemistry of sexual arousal and how our history of previous sexual experiences plays a part in every new sexual experience we have. To explore the emotional aspect of our feelings around sexuality in more depth, it is useful to go back to some basics, to understand the build-ing blocks behind our more complex emotions.

There are four primary emotions expressed in the extreme by human infants, and, most often, more moderately by adults.

- Ecstasy → Joy
- Rage → Anger
- Terror → Fear
- Misery → Sorrow

They are called primary emotions because they can be experienced by all of us and we can recognise them in others. They are reflexes, triggered in response to something or someone. They are processed first through the memory centres of the limbic system in the brain, reacting with a flood of neurochemicals, activating the autonomous nervous system, and causing physiological effects.

Let us take a moment to consider how we know which emotion we are feeling. Usually, there is a combination of physical sensations and reactions and specific thoughts. It is useful to notice and accept the somatic experiences of each emotion, and to separate our thoughts. Anger will increase our heart rate and trigger muscle tension, causing a more firm body stance. Joy and happiness is often a welcome feel-ing: waves of pleasure in the body, excitement, and anticipation. Fear might induce a desire to retreat, a tensing of muscles in the upper body, and thinking about what to do. Sorrow might produce a pain in the heart, the release of tears, feelings of sadness, and thoughts of being rejected and abandoned.

The survival circuits are just that: necessary to our wellbeing. Fight tells us we are in danger and need to act. When we show anger and someone takes us seriously, and perhaps offers acts of correction, we feel cared about. Fear indicates a need to get away and requires actions to re-establish safety. If we appear frightened and someone takes action to increase our sense of security, we feel looked after. Panic is an expression of sorrow and loss of attachment to an other. If we express our sadness and are met with acts of compassion by another, such as empathy or a cuddle, we can feel soothed. The social-ising brain circuits introduced in the "Brain" section (caring, curiosity, and play) often elicit feelings of joy: vitality and expressions of plea-sure. When we show our joy and another responds by smiling at us, we feel seen and witnessed.

Because emotions are processed through the memory centres, our experience of them and what we think as a consequence will be related to our unique histories. We learn through experience after experience being laid down, building a picture, our story of how the world operates. This will also develop according to the responses elicited from our carers in response to our emotions as children. If our emotional requests were responded to kindly, we will more comfort-ably accept our emotionality and that of others. For example, some people might feel comfortable being sexual or showing this aspect of themselves in front of someone else, while others might feel deeply ashamed about this happening.

We may have been taught, and still think or believe, that certain emotions are signs of "weakness" or are inappropriate to show. We have cultural stereotypes that women may show tears but not rage, and that men may show anger but not fear. What we *think* about what we are feeling and, therefore, judge how we think we should behave, is often what distresses us, rather than which emotions we are actually feeling. We could utilise our emotional response as a baseline reaction: we will either feel happy with what is happening, or not. Either we are all right, or we are sad, angry, or frightened. Our emotions, rather than being problematic for us, can become an easy, clear indicator if we consider their purpose. Their universality could be seen as a non-verbal method of communication for and between humans, their expression as an attempt to elicit a specific empathic response in others. Understanding the purpose of different emotions, helps us to be clearer about our own responses, and what we might want. It also helps us to understand what others might want from us in response to their expressions of emotion, which is vital for good relationships.

Our four basic emotions are an instinctive reflex from the brain, with identifiable physical responses in us, including facial responses, body postures, and tone and pitch of voice. We then use our frontal lobes to reflect and assess and decide how to react. This sounds simplistic and, on some level, it is. By becoming more conscious about how we think about our emotions and how we use them, we can acknowledge that how we think actually has the biggest impact on how we behave. As discussed in the "Mind" section, what and how we think is also correlated to our past experiences, as well as our social and cultural beliefs. We can evaluate and update our values and belief systems and so change and adapt our thinking. By accepting our basic reactivity, understanding and having compassion for our own personal history, we can more consciously take responsibility for how we behave now as an adult.

There are also more complex emotions, such as confusion, frustration, disappointment, jealousy, envy, pride, embarrassment, sympathy, and gratitude. Frustration may be a combination of anger and sadness, confusion, wanting to do one thing and thinking we should do something else. Complex emotions are connected to our perceptions of our emotions, to us as social beings, and what others might expect of us or think about us. Our feelings and emotions about sexuality are deeply affected by our cultural responses to sexuality and attitudes of sexual shame.

The more clearly we can identify the different aspects of our feelings of sexual arousal, of sexual desire, our reactions from the back brain, the somatic responses of our body, our thinking and, now, the specifics of our emotions, the more we understand and can consciously choose how we might want to act in response. Within this model, all are probably happening, and all affecting and being affected by the others. It may be useful to consider which of these aspects are most easily identifiable and which you struggle more to comprehend.

Exercise   Your feelings

Read over what you have written about the earlier exercises on 'Emotional awareness', about the primary emotions of anger, fear, sadness, and joy. How comfortable or uncomfortable do you feel experiencing each emotion?

Think about the more complex emotions of disappointment or frustration, for example. How easy or difficult is it for you to manage these feelings?

Consider which feelings and emotions were easily expressed and allowed during your childhood or not allowed and discouraged. How have your early life experiences affected how you are as an adult? Identify any ways of responding to your feelings you would like to change and think about how you could do that.

Think about your feelings and experiences of joy, happiness, and excitement. How were these treated during your early life? Consider how has this may have affected how you feel about your sexuality now.

Shame and sexuality

In Britain, we have a culture of shame around our emotions. Being emotional is often seen as a weakness and being "rational" as a strength. If we have feelings, we are encouraged to suppress and hide our somatic reactions; displays of emotion are often criticised as a sign of immaturity. Bradshaw's work on shame (2005) identifies different levels of shame from mild to toxic, and explores how this plays out within family systems. Within the homeodynamic model, human experience of ourselves and of others is a combination of a reaction in the back brain, a series of somatic experiences and emotions, and a capacity to reflect on all of these and make some choices about how we will behave in response. The point is that our feelings and emotions are what we base our rationale, our thinking, on. To believe some aspects of our humanity are more important or valuable is to deny a large part of being human. This general shaming around emotions contributes to our experience of our sexuality as shaming, as our sexual selves include displaying our emotions, feeling sensations in our body, thinking sexual thoughts, and, often, behaving in sexual ways. Tomkins (cited in Nathanson, 1992) believed that one reason we have a social shaming of sexuality is because there is no other human activity that so exposes what is normally private (our bodies). We are, therefore, made capable of embarrassment by nearly everything associated with sexual performance. When we are being sexual with others, we give up our social rules to modulate displays of emotion.

Kaufman and Raphael (1996) see our current gender ideology as hetero-normative, with unspoken rules about power and control in male to female relationships: that men should exercise power and dominate over women; that women should not exercise power and should submit to men. They considered that one reason for shaming of sexual minorities is in relation to breaking such cultural rules about expressions of emotions and of power. Social and cultural homophobia can contribute to internalised homophobia.

In Tomkins's work on affects, he identified disgust and shame as also being seen as "negative" reactions. He adds "dismell", which is a reaction to aromas or odours, where the upper lip and the cheeks become raised and the nose bridge wrinkled. Smell is a powerful sense for humans, probably because there is only one synaptic jump from the olfactory bulb in the nose to the limbic system. It is known to trigger strong memories quickly. We have a cultural dismell to our natural smells, especially in relation to ourselves sexually, with many products aimed at disguising or hiding them. This is strange, as pheromones, smell aromas that we release and respond to, are part of our human sexual responses.

Disgust is described as ranging from *contemptuous* (scornful, disrespectful, or sarcastic) to *disgusted* (revolted, repelled, or put off by), where the lower lip becomes lowered and protruded. *Shame* includes feeling exposed, embarrassed, and self-conscious, or, more intensely, as *humiliation* (feeling mortified, alienated, and disgraced), expressed with the head lowered, downcast eyes, and vasodilation of the face and skin resulting in blushing.

Shame can be seen as the principle source of our conscience, that something is not all right between us and another person. Shame is often taken to be information about the self, but Lee (2008) says it is information about what is happening in the relational field, that is, between an individual and someone else. He says it is an attempt to protect when we know, or imagine, that there is not enough support in the relational field for us to be accepted. It is about the quality or lack of reception in the relationship (being accepted, acceptable). Shame helps us to keep the problem (of not being received) hidden and, therefore, not to show our vulnerability or distress.

Shame can be seen as a necessary survival regulator; it protects us against rejection (not being received/welcomed). Humans need relationships; as infants, we would die if not "in relationship" with someone to care for us. Kaufman and Raphael (1996) say that without the experience of shame, there would be nothing to alert us to ruptures in our relationships. So, on an evolutionary level, shame provides protection and safety; we hide and withdraw, brush down, and achieve space in which to collect ourselves so that we can go out again and try to be received by someone else. This keeps our desire and curiosity intact, and our human need to stay in relationship.

Where there is shame, there is yearning or desire. We are only capable of experiencing shame if we care about the connection: what we want and/or who we want it with. We cannot feel shame if there is nothing to lose. Equally, the greater the importance, the more intense the experience of shame will be. When we are not received in relationship, this undermines our confidence and sense of self; we become unsure of what is going on "between" us. This can lead to self-shaming, where, instead of seeing that the other person is not the one to meet our yearning and seeking someone else who might do so, we believe we should not have wanted it in the first place. We might have internalised negative beliefs about our rights to have needs and desires, and our rights to have these needs met in relationship. We might close down these needs and hide physically and emotionally from ourselves as well as from others. Healing shame requires us to go back to the original yearning, what it is we wanted, and to feel and process the pain and disappointment of not having that yearning met. We can then reclaim or moderate our desire, and then, again, ask for that yearning to be met.

We can have many reactions to shame. We might become fearful, distressed, or enraged; all act to shield the exposed self. Kaufman and Raphael suggest we have four main counter shaming strategies: withdrawal, attack self, avoidance, and attack other (Figure 17). They say all are an avoidance of intimacy, of eye contact; we avoid the gaze of others.

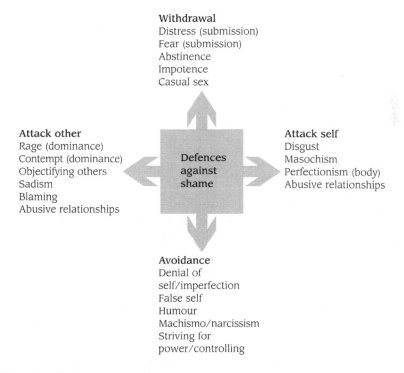

Figure 17.   Defences against shame.

Exercise   Sexual shame

Most of us probably experience some degree of shame about our sexuality, given our cultures. Think about your beliefs in connection with the different aspects listed below and indicate whether they make you feel proud or ashamed.

Beliefs about	Proud	Ashamed
Sex		
Sexuality		
Sensuality		
Your childhood		
Sexual history		
Your teenage sexual history		
Your body		
Your body image		
Your sexual identity		
Your relationship to sexuality now		
Your current sexual behaviour		
Your sexual relationships		
Your sexual fantasies		
Your creativity		
Your passion		

Review your list. Overall, do you predominately feel proud or ashamed of your sexuality? Choose one issue you feel ashamed about. Consider whether you want to reclaim a sense of self-esteem about your choices or preferences, or whether your shame is an indicator that you may want to change your beliefs or behaviour in some way.

Pain or pleasure

If shame is an indication of a rupture in the relational field, what might this mean for us in an evaluation of sexual shame? Our sexual feelings can be triggered by a sensory experience of someone else (a sight, sound, or smell), or a memory of a sexual encounter. However our arousal is triggered, it often results in a desire to be sexual with an other. Whether that desire is to touch and be touched, to cuddle or to kiss, to penetrate or be penetrated, it is often something we want to do to, or with, someone else. Even when we are being sexual with ourselves, we are being in a relationship of sorts: we are responding physically to a feeling, a desire, a sensation, with a choice to behave sexually.

To explore the relational field of our sexuality, let us go back and consider the fundamental relational needs of humans and vital developmental stages in our formative years. Hendrix (1995) outlines a psychosocial journey of the self from birth to teenage, with six identifiable stages, each with a primary behaviour. Figure 18 shows how we build these psychosocial skills that lead to an integrated sense of responsibility to self and to society.

He believed that when a child is allowed and supported through each stage successfully, this would lead to a specific developmental achievement. Transition through all stages will allow a development of responsibility to self and to society, an acceptance of our needs, a fundamental belief in our right to have these needs, and our trust that they can, and mostly will, be met. When our needs are not met, we might believe essentially that somehow we should not have these needs and feel shame in relation to them. If this is the case, what impact miught this have on how we feel about ourselves sexually?

Age	Developmental task	Developmental behaviour	Psychosocial skills
Birth – 18 months	ATTACHMENT	Reaching	Emotional security
18 months – 3 years	EXPLORATION	Exploring	Differentiation & intact curiosity
3 – 4 years	IDENTITY	Asserting	Secure sense of self
4 – 7 years	COMPETENCE	Competing	Sense of personal power to achieve
7 – 13 years	CONCERN	Sympathising	Concern for others
13 – 19 years	INTIMACY	Integrating	Intact sexuality Ability to love

Figure 18.   The Hendrix psychosocial stages of development.

Exercise   Personal power

Think about the stages outlined in Figure 18 and described in the pages above.
Write a bit about how they were supported or undermined during your childhood.

Attachment
Touch and holding
Exploration
Belonging, being different
Identity
The right to choose
Competence
Affirmation of worth
Concern
Care for others
Intimacy
Relationship with others

Reflect on how this has affected you as an adult. During which phases were you
encouraged and supported and in which were you hampered? How has this
affected how you feel towards yourself and towards others?

Playing with fire

How do we get to play with our sexuality as adults? It is said that
we now live in a highly sexualised culture, but do we truly celebrate our human sexual pleasure and feel sexual self-esteem? Between
our historic religious anti-sex dictates, parents not feeling comfortable
to educate children about their sexuality and sexual relationships,
and school's sex education focusing on reproduction, there has been
a social and cultural void of information or celebration of human
sexuality. People want to know more; many are rightly curious about
this exciting yet shamed aspect of being human. The amount of
pornography has exploded in the past decade and stepped in to fill
that gap. With the advent of broadband Internet, access has become
easily available through the privacy of your own home or mobile
phone.

Pornography is still largely a male preserve and is marketed and
consumed specifically to trigger sexual arousal, through the sight of
images and the sight and sound of film and video. Opinions about
pornography cross a broad spectrum between those who promote it
and those who think it should be banned. The arguments for seem to

be that it is educational, helps to liberate us sexually, and that it offers a world of fun and fantasy for adults. The arguments against seem to focus mostly on pornography aimed at heterosexuals, which some claim is misogynistic, promotes sexual selfishness in men (Boyle, 2007), and has seriously lowered our standards for sexual interactions to nothing more than "ejaculating over increasingly humiliating acts of penetration" (Maltz, 2010). Banyard (2010) calls it "a sexier form of sexism". There seems to be less controversy for gay men; maybe gay pornography depicts more what gay men want to do to and with each other. Equally, pornography made for lesbians (that is really made for them rather than "girl on girl action" made for straight men) seems to be more acceptable.

Pornography is said to have played a role in reducing our cultural shame about sexuality by explicitly acknowledging a range of sexual behaviours and giving people permission to experiment sexually. Some women feel liberated to own a more potent sexual life. Pornography shows women as being just as hungry for sex as men, just as desirous of pleasure and fun, way beyond the "dutiful wife". The Centre for Sex Positive Culture (2011) has a mission to "inspire and assist volunteers to produce experiential events where members can explore their sexual interests in a physically and emotionally safe environment". Some women working in the sex industry feel empowered to earn a better living (than from doing most other jobs), and are supporting children or taking themselves through college. Many women working on the web feel empowered to just "switch off" anyone they do not want to deal with.

A collection of research from academic specialists in this field was edited by Attwood (2010). She argues that contemporary pornography "challenges normative constructions of gender and sexuality" and "represents a cultural shift towards new public forms of talking about sex". She comments that some research shows that pornography, rather than producing any measurable "effect", is experienced in a variety of ways by consumers. For example, many have discerning opinions, take ethical positions on the pornography debate, and act as responsible parents in terms of the media their children encounter. Surprisingly little research had actually been conducted until McKee, Albury, and Lumby (2008). They surveyed over 1,000 consumers of pornography in Australia about their perceived negative and positive effects of using pornography.

- Fifty-nine per cent of respondents thought pornography had had a very positive or a positive effect on their attitudes towards sexuality.
- Thirty-five per cent felt it had had no effect.
- Seven per cent thought it had a negative effect or a large negative effect.

The main positive effects, in order of reporting, were: making consumers less repressed about sex; making them more open-minded about sex; increasing tolerance of other people's sexualities; giving pleasure to consumers; providing educational insights; sustaining sexual interest in long-term relationships; making consumers more attentive to a partner's sexual desires; helping consumers find an identity or community; helping them to talk to their partners about sex. The most common negative effects cited in this study were that pornography led consumers to objectify people; caused them to have unrealistic sexual expectations; caused relationship problems; caused loss of interest in sex; led to addiction.

One of the main critiques made of pornography is about actual harm. Banyard (2010) claims that eighty-nine per cent of scenes in mainstream pornography depict aggressive acts, nearly all directed at women. Walter (2010) believes that pornography devalues our sexual experience into brutalised penetration, where men are encouraged to see women as sexual objects, and women encouraged to focus on their sexual allure rather than their own sexual pleasure. In 2007 Boyle made a submission to the Equal Opportunities Committee of the Scottish Parliament on the impact of pornography. She addressed issues of harm in heterosexual porn:

- harmful production practices: the discomfort, pain, or physical injuries sustained through posing or performing, and the defamation of women who have appeared in pornography productions;
- the depiction of unsafe sexual practices;
- representations of harm with the text itself, including:
  - the objectification of women into types (such as "Asian", "Teen"), or parts (such as "Big Breasts");
  - the derogatory language used, such as "bitch", "filthy whore", "dirty cunt";

o   scenes of humiliation, with twenty-five per cent depicting violence.

It would be useful to move beyond the pro-pornography and anti-pornography stances. If we were to acknowledge the benefits and advantages, and to review and address its potential disadvantages, we could consider what forms of sexually explicit material might be socially advantageous. Censorship or criminalisation often carry a repressive agenda and seem to focus primarily on pathologising minorities. The International Prostitutes Collective (accessed 6 January 2012) campaigns for the decriminalisation of prostitution, for sex workers' right to recognition and safety, and for financial alternatives so that no one is forced into prostitution by poverty.

On an educational level, most bodies displayed in pornography are incredibly unrealistic: for example, abnormally large penises which are always erect. There are rarely views of flaccid penises or foreskins, what they look like, or their more realistic size.

Breasts are large and silicone enhanced and vulvas look as if they belong to a prepubescent girl. The focus on penetration in pornography encourages the myth that "real sex" is penetration and undermines the fact that the clitoris is women's sexual organ. The depiction of women being orgasmic through the penetration of various orifices is also blatantly unrealistic. The focus on sexual acts rarely addresses safer sex, or educates people about negotiating sexual encounters or relationship. A recent campaign in America, spearheaded by the AIDS Healthcare Foundation, has resulted in a law in Los Angeles requiring that condoms are used during pornographic film shots. The law was fought by production companies, who are threatening to leave the city to work elsewhere (Papenfuss, 2012).

Pornography has played a role in challenging our cultural shame about sex, and we are more open in talking about sex and our needs and desires. But have we flipped the coin to merely the opposite, shamelessness, rather than creating conscious sexual self-esteem? Attwood (2010) noted people reporting contradictory feelings of being simultaneously attracted and repulsed by pornography. In her comments about harm, Boyle (2007) said many users reported feeling ambivalence and shame. For men, this can act out as discord in their relationships with women partners, friends, or peers. For women, this might mean a contradiction between the urge to appear sexy and that of wanting to experience sexual pleasure. Women were also more likely to have confusing feelings about enjoying the pornography, while also having empathy with the social, emotional, and physical plight of the female performers. Boynton (2011) points out that some women seem much more anxious about the issues of body image and female attractiveness in pornography than they do about issues of sexual violence.

Many years ago, Nathanson (1992) commented on how our advertising and entertainment industries actually display what he identified as defences against shame. This is probably more common now, with magazines, soap operas, and reality television programmes showing "attack self" attitudes through perfectionism and body fascism, and "attack others" through the ridicule and humiliation of celebrities, or of those who think that they have "talent". The viewer can look into the eyes of others; they can stare and not have their gaze returned. The object of their gaze cannot look back and see into their eyes, so there is no risk of shaming. Within Nathanson's model, shame is a relational experience: we only feel shame in response to not being acceptable to the "other". Pornography provides anonymity, for both the sex worker and the consumer. Ultimately, Nathanson believes pornography is also a shame-based phenomenon. It also shows some evidence of avoidance and withdrawal from sexual encounters with real, imperfect people, and of "attack self and other" through its focus on "degradation and body punishing penetration" and language that is routinely aggressive and derogatory (Dines 2010).

Within the homeodynamic model of health, there are other concerns about which neurochemicals pornography triggers and what impacts this might have on the "survival" and the "socialising" brain circuits.

The survival circuit comprises

- *fight*: danger, need to take action;
- *flight*: need to get away, withdraw;
- *panic*: abandonment, loss, separation distress.

The socialising circuit is composed of

- *caring*: our capacity to have empathy and look after other people;
- *curiosity*: our interest in others and the world around us;
- *play and physical contact*: our need for touch and fun with others.

Maltz (2010) says pornography acts like a designer drug, aimed at hitting the reward system, offering novelty, excitement, escape, and then relaxation through orgasm. It is ingested through the eyes and ears, not through touching or being touched by another. This can lead to a loss of sensuality and less oxytocin during the process of arousal, leaving it more adrenalised, more likely to activate the survival circuits of the brain and the primary emotions of anger, fear, and sadness. (This is obviously less so when pornography is used as part of sex play with another.) Pornography activates plenty of adrenalin to fuel the arousal, dopamine to motivate us (which triggers the curiosity circuit), and endorphins, which reduce feelings of pain. At climax, there are surges of serotonin and prolactin, which make us feel good, and of oxytocin, which promotes feelings of love and bonding. Of the socialising circuits, the need for play and physical contact includes a need for touch. If there is no real person to touch, could an attachment become formed with the pornography itself, leading to a higher propensity for addiction? Carnes, Delmonico, and Griffin (2007) discuss in depth the role of pornography in the increasing rates of sexual compulsivity.

What is missing from the socialising circuits is caring. McGilchrist (2009) argues that objectification and the consumerism of sex utilise left-brain activity. He says the right brain is embodied, in touch with ourselves and the reality of interaction with others. The left brain decontextualises our experiences, turning us away, in his opinion, from what most defines us as human beings: our capacity for empathy. Mainstream pornography does seem to promote a lack of empathy about the reality of the experience for the women sex workers. A recent survey (Farley, Bindel, & Golding, 2009) indicated that many of the male respondents were aware of pimping, trafficking, and other coercive control over those in massage parlours and brothels (where most sex was bought), but few did anything about it. Attitudes normalising rape were common among this group of men. Twenty-four per cent asserted that the concept of rape simply does not apply to women in prostitution: once he pays, the customer is entitled to engage in *any act he chooses* with the woman he buys.

In the past, the "sex industry" was a business with its main aim to make as much money as possible from the desires people have to be sexually aroused; it is said to turn over ninety-seven billion dollars a year. There was no particular concern about the health and safety or working conditions of its employees. But it seems this is changing.

Many people use pornography as part of masturbation. Most people discover this form of self-soothing around eight years old (Hite, 1994) and most have felt or experienced shame about it. This can lead to a sense that it should be done in secret, and as quickly as possible. Using pornography to induce orgasm as quickly as possible avoids the plateau phase of the arousal process, the phase that necessitates consciousness of being highly aroused.

Erotica is becoming more focused on the conscious enjoyment of pleasure; it can offer a "sex positive" vision and has the potential to affirm sexual diversity and marginalised sexualities. Humans feel sexual desire and sometimes want to masturbate, to have their arousal stimulated by the sight and sounds of someone/something sexy. They become aroused and feel pleasure from seeing someone else show their sexual pleasure. Part of our gift of sexuality is to be able to pleasure ourselves, for fun, for relaxation, or for self-soothing. We are moving into an era where sexuality can be celebrated and played with, using sexually explicit material and sex toys and games, either alone or within relationships (see Carrellas, 2007; Sprinkle, 2011). Attwood (2010) says there are now many more small producers alongside the big companies and more people (particularly women) making pornography to their own tastes. An indicator of sexual self-esteem is that we feel comfortable with, and proud of, our sexual arousal and sexual experiences. The question is not, perhaps, whether pornography is good or bad, but, rather, what the quality is of what we are consuming and whether it is enhancing our sexual self-esteem or maintaining an ethos of sexual shame.

Exercise   Passionate play

Explore your relationship to sexual play. Do you like to play sexually, and, if so, how do you do this? Do you like how you play, or is there something you would like to change? If you don't like how you play or how often you play, how could you change this? For example, do you make enough time and space in your life to play; are you playing in the way that you really want to?

Research online or go to visit a sex shop. You may want to go with a friend or a lover. There are some for heterosexuals, some aimed at gay men, and some for women only. Explore what sort of toys are out there for sex play and see what you think and feel about it? Make some choices about what you like and what you don't.

Notice your first reactions, especially any strong reactions. Is there some attraction along with any repulsion? Explore whether there is shame about what you "should or shouldn't" want and consider whether you want to challenge these first reactions. Discuss with some others what they think and why.

Sexual addiction

Much has been written about sexual addiction in recent years and there is still controversy about its definition, particularly whether it is another way of pathologising certain sexual lifestyles and an increasing liberalisation of our cultural attitudes to sex. As with addiction to any substance, sexual addiction is about using sex as a defence against feelings, which return, perhaps more intensely after the high, leading to a low. This can lead to a cycle of increasing "acting out" behaviour. Sex is no longer fun, but has become a coping mechanism to regulate emotional life, now connected with survival rather than pleasure. As the behaviours are a deflection activity, they are not satiating, leading to an increase—hence the cycle.

Carnes (2001) defines sexual addiction as "a pathological relationship with a mood-altering chemical/experience". He believes this leads to a four-step cycle of compulsivity that intensifies with each repetition:

1. Preoccupation: the trance or mood wherein the addicts' minds are obsessively engrossed with thoughts of sex and in search of sexual stimulation.
2. Ritualisation: the addicts' own special routines that lead up to the sexual behaviour. The ritual intensifies the preoccupation, adding arousal and excitement.
3. Compulsive sexual behaviour: the sexual acts, which are the end goal of preoccupation and ritualisation. Sex addicts may feel unable to control or stop this behaviour.
4. Despair: the feeling of utter hopelessness addicts have about their behaviour and powerlessness.

Addiction may be one of the "defences against shame" outlined by Kaufman and Raphael earlier, but, sadly, it only compounds the problem. Along with the attractions, there can be an associated repulsion. Shame about the acting out can lead to greater attempts to control behaviour, which often fails and leads to more feeling bad, leading to beginning the cycle again. Martin-Sperry (2004) likens this to the eating disorder, bulimia, with a repetitive pattern of sexual binging and guilt and a searching for comfort and relief. She also includes sexual anorexia; in the same way as food, sex can become part of a bargaining tool, to be withheld for power and control. She discusses the histories of abuse and shame common for those with such issues.

Goodman (1998) argues it is not so much the sexual behaviours themselves that define addiction, but the relationship to them: first, recurrent failure to control the behaviour and, second, continuation of the behaviour despite significant harmful consequences. Consequences can include social, academic, financial, psychological, or physical problems such as sexually transmitted infections or getting into dangerous situations. This can lead to a neglect of important social relationships, like family or friends, or of professional responsibilities, or recreational activities. Partner relationships can break down or suffer chaos and emotional pain. There can be a longing for relationships with intimacy, good communication, and healthy sexuality.

Time loss is a major factor in sexual compulsivity; inordinate amounts of time may be spent in obtaining sex, being sexual, or recovering from sexual experiences. Acting out can affect work performance and energy levels, leading to losing a job and/or social reputation or status. It can lead to isolation through focusing on gaining sexual opportunities rather than social or relationship opportunities. The consequences can also include mental health issues such as loneliness, fear of getting caught out/paranoia, being discovered, anxiety, fear of ageing, and life transitions becoming more challenging.

Weiss (2005) challenges the twelve-step addiction model, arguing that it pathologises gay lifestyles. He offers a more sex affirmative approach to addressing compulsivity that might be detrimental in some ways. He defines sexual addiction in terms of what healthy sexuality is not:

- obsession;
- compulsion;
- trance-like-states;
- repeated poor judgement for one's physical, emotional, and legal safety.

He believes many factors contribute to sexual compulsivity, including low self-esteem, a need for validation and affection, using sex as an escape from depression or to relieve stress. He sees factors such as childhood sexual abuse or other traumatic life events, relationship breakdown, pornography, and drug or alcohol abuse as triggers to sexually acting out. He says that gay men might be more vulnerable to sexual compulsivity due to cultural shame, internalised homophobia, or poor body image.

Kort (2011) says that some issues that present in couple therapy can be signs of compulsivity. For example, where online pornography use interferes with primary relationships, such as minimising or lying about time or money spent, or not considering online "affairs" to be a possible violation of partnership commitments. Signs of co-addiction can include beliefs that sex is the most important sign of love in the relationship, covering up for partners' behaviour or related financial or legal problems.

Nathanson (1992) discusses sexual addiction by looking at the similarities and differences between food and sexual appetite. He says when we are hungry or thirsty, our desire to eat or drink is satiated before the nutrients are absorbed by the body: somehow, knowing we are in the act of eating/drinking satiates us. The nature of sexual arousal, however, is that, once aroused or interested, we usually want more, more touch, more stimulation, until we have had enough. But what is enough? The arousal circuits described in Part III remind us of the importance of the plateau phase. Once arousal has begun and the sexual charge has built the excitation, then it levels out to plateau, which extends to the brink of orgasm. This involves relaxation and letting go to enjoying a heightened state of sexual arousal.

Basson (2001), in her circular model of sexual arousal, refers to a subjective experience of sexual arousal and sexual desire, including emotional intimacy, emotional and physical satisfaction, as well as biological and psychological factors. In order to enjoy the plateau, we need to be free of shame, be content to experience ourselves as being sexually aroused, and be willing to be seen. We need to have a sense of what is "enough", of what is satiating to us. This will depend very much on how we progressed through the developmental phases outlined above: attachment, exploration, identity, competence, and concern; were we able to successfully integrate these phases, to develop an intact sexuality and an ability to be intimate and to love? Gerhardt (2004) describes how emotional deprivation in early childhood alters dopamine pathways, particularly in the limbic system, increasing greedy and impulsive behaviours, and providing a disposition to addiction.

Kaufman and Raphael (1996) argue that we can become addicted to excitement itself. The chemicals released in the body during the high of acting out sexually include internal mood enhancers such as adrenalin and dopamine. They believe substances are less likely to be addictive when they are used to enhance *positive* affects, as described above, and more likely to be addictive when they are used to reduce or sedate *negative* affects. In their opinion, addiction is most likely

- when the substance is transformed into an end in itself;
- when an absence of substance leads to panic;
- where the substance becomes the only relief from panic.

"Panic", within the homeodynamic model, is about loss of attachment, sadness and grief about loss of relationship. It is easy to see how unresolved attachment and developmental issues play a role in addictions and compulsivity: the urge to reach out, to be held and touched, to have physical and emotional needs satiated. Using sex as an activity to fulfil attachment needs will only work if there is an attachment. That does not mean that we should only have sex in "relationships", but it helps if we are in "relationship" with ourselves by being embodied and consciously embarking on our sexual activities. Using the exercises in this book can help to highlight what relationship we want with our sexuality and encourage us to make more conscious choices about our sexual beliefs and sexual behaviour that we can feel proud about.

Exercise   Challenging compulsion

Write a list of any compulsive behaviour that you have. Choose one that you would like to change, or at least explore in more depth.

Sit for a while in your safe space and take some time to relax. Think more about what you like and don't like about this particular behaviour. Consider whether the compulsivity is connected to the behaviour not satiating your needs, or whether it has become a habit. Try not to censor what is evoked for you, but allow any thoughts, body sensations, memories, and feelings and notice what they are.

Write something about each of the following and then reflect on what you have written:

My thoughts about this behaviour are . . .

Thinking about this behaviour evokes the following body sensations . . .

The memories that are triggered include . . .

How I am feeling is . . .

Now think back to the last time you acted out the behaviour you are exploring and take your attention to the hours and minutes just beforehand. What were you thinking and feeling then?

Can you identify exactly what outcome you wanted to happen, what need did you want met? Did you get that need met so that you felt completely satiated? If not, what aspect was not met?

Do you feel any shame about what you wanted? If so, think about why. Is this need something you were discouraged from wanting as a child? Is there something about what you are doing or how you are trying to get this need met that is not working for you? Try to identify what exactly is not working for you.

Now think about something that you do that leaves you feeling satiated. Describe in detail what it feels like to feel satiated, how does that feel in your body, your thoughts, and your emotions?

Think about how you could change any aspect of the behaviour you have explored in this exercise so you could alter your relationship to it.

Sexual violence

If you are someone who has experienced sexual violence as an adult or childhood sexual abuse, you might find reading this section evokes feelings of anger or distress. Please go back to the beginning of the book and re-read the exercise "Applying the brakes" and consider whether you are in the right time and space to continue. You might want to skip this section and come back to it another time.

Sexual violence is still a huge problem for many people, with estimates that one in four women have experienced rape or attempted rape (Rape Crisis, 2004–2012). The statistic that three in twenty men are affected by sexual violence is almost certainly a huge under-estimation, as many male rape victims are extremely reluctant to report such attacks to the police (Mankind, 2011). The impact of sexual violence and sexual abuse is devastating. It affects not only victims in terms of physical and mental health, but also affects their families, communities, and the wider society. Sexual violence against women also includes female genital mutilation (FGM), crimes in the name of honour, and trafficking. The value of the global trade in women as commodities for sex industries is estimated to be between seven and twelve billion dollars annually. Women are trafficked for the purpose of sexual exploitation to, from, and through every region in the world, using methods that some say have become new forms of slavery (Hughes, 2000). Rape and the sexual assault of both males and females have always been, and continue to be, a strategy in war.

There are many more rapes and sexual assaults reported in the British Crime Surveys and to rape crisis services than are formally reported to the police. Some recent facts:

- In the year to March 2011, there were 15,940 rapes reported to the police in England and Wales, with twenty four per cent of cases leading to conviction or caution (BBC News, 2011).
- Nationally, the majority of reported rapes are from under eighteens; in London, this accounts for nearly half of all reported rapes (Family Lives, 2011).
- More than one third of all rapes recorded by the police are committed against children under sixteen years of age (Department of Health, 2010).
- One in three teenage girls tells of sexual abuse by their boyfriends (Carter, 2009).
- A government report (Department of Health, 2010) claimed that sexual violence or abuse against children represents a major public health and social welfare problem within UK society, affecting twenty-one per cent of girls and eleven per cent of boys under sixteen years old.
- In 2008–2009, ChildLine, the twenty-four-hour confidential helpline for children, counselled 12,268 children for sexual violence and abuse, representing a forty-two per cent increase over three years (National Society for the Prevention of Cruelty to Children (NSPCC), 2009).

Changes to the 1956 Sexual Offences Act in 1994 made the rape of a man an equal crime to the rape of a woman (prior to that time, only the non-consensual penetration of a woman by a penis of a man other than her husband was considered as rape; any other assaults were covered by the lesser crime of "sexual assault"). Further updates to the Sexual Offences Act mean that the different types of sexual assault have been defined. The Sexual Offences Act 2003 replaces the 1956 Act and redefines as follows.

- Rape to include penetration of the mouth or anus, and a new offence of sexual assault by penetration, covers acts involving the insertion of objects or body parts other than the penis. This includes assaults against males and females and also "marital rape" between co-habiting or separated intimate partners.
- Sexual assault—any kind of intentional sexual touching of somebody else without their consent. It includes touching any part of their body, clothed or unclothed, either with their body or with an object.
- Causing a person to engage in a sexual activity without consent—any kind of sexual activity without consent. For instance, it would apply to an abuser who makes their victim engage in masturbation.
- Government guidance (Working Together to Safeguard Children), defines child sexual abuse as forcing or enticing a child or young person to take part in sexual activities, including prostitution, whether or not the child is aware of what is happening. The activities might involve physical contact, including penetrative or non-penetrative acts. They might include non-contact activities, such as involving children in looking at, or in the production of, sexual online images, watching sexual activities, or encouraging children to behave in sexually inappropriate ways.
- Sexual bullying: any bullying behaviour, whether physical or non-physical, that is based on a person's sexuality or gender. It is when sexuality or gender is used as a weapon by boys or girls towards other boys or girls—although it is more commonly directed at girls. It can be carried out to a person's face, behind their back, or through the use of technology.

Parentlineplus (2011) say there is evidence that sexual bullying of young people is increasing, with a twenty per cent rise in the number of children being given court orders and warnings for sex offences by the Youth Justice Board. A survey of nearly 2,000 teenage girls in 2006 revealed an abusive undercurrent within much of their early sexual experimentation, which left them feeling dirty, ashamed/guilty, worried/insecure, angry, powerless, and frightened (Farmer, 2009):

- forty-five per cent had been groped against their wishes;
- fifty-six per cent of unwanted sexual experiences occurred for the first time when girls were under fourteen;

- fifty-one per cent of unwanted sexual experiences occurred more than once.

The new legislation has gone some way to identify the real scope of sexual violence, but we still retain a cultural ambivalence to the subject: on the one hand, we consider rape and sexual assault as serious crimes, and, on the other, we still maintain beliefs that victims are to blame. A poll for Amnesty in 2005 found that

- a third of people believe women who flirt are partially responsible for being raped;
- a quarter of those asked said that they thought a woman was partially or totally responsible for being raped if she was wearing sexy or revealing clothing;
- more than one in five held the same view if a woman has many sexual partners;
- around one in twelve people believed that a woman was totally responsible for being raped if she has many sexual partners;
- more than a quarter of people (thirty per cent) said that a woman was partially or totally responsible for being raped if she was drunk.

Nathanson (1992) discussed our cultural ambivalence to sexual violence when writing about the social impacts of shame twenty years ago. He commented then on trends in cruelty in sexually violent films, in what he called a "cultural explosion of the Macho script". He saw this as a shame defence (attack others), where anger and fear trigger excitement. He said that what is being produced is "more humiliating, more deadly, more violent, and more graphically rendered than at any time in our history", and reminds us that such things are happening in real life. We certainly still have many films and video games that glorify violence and sexualised violence, both of which are a huge part of our entertainment industry.

Being a victim of sexual violence or abuse is a risk factor for the development of serious mental health difficulties, including post traumatic stress disorder, clinical depression, generalised anxiety disorder, and separation anxiety disorder. Many survivors attempt suicide or turn to substance abuse. Other long-term problems include guilt and self-blame, low self-esteem and negative self-image, problems with intimacy, compulsions, or sexual difficulties. Sexual violence is an assault against the body and the mind and it invades a person's integrity. It sullies an aspect of them, their sexuality, which is supposed to be associated with freedom and pleasure, not with pain, fear, or confusion. Figure 19 shows some of the issues within the homeodynamic model. Many of the topics could easily be placed in more than one section, as they could have a physical and a psychological component, and, as discussed earlier, all aspects might trigger, or be triggered by, other issues. This list is not exhaustive.

Added complications for male survivors include sexual stereotypes that men are supposed to be strong and able to take care of themselves, and myths that only gay men are raped. In 1999, the Royal College of Nursing Congress (Survivors UK, 2012) called for the government to address urgently the lack of services for, and information on, male rape. They claim that some of the long-term effects of sexual abuse are related to the development of gender identity.

Brain	Mind
■ Post-traumatic stress activating the limbic system ■ Dis-regulated neurochemicals ■ Agitation to the nervous system ■ Fusion or confusion between the reward and punishment circuits ■ Unwanted or inappropriate arousal ■ Flashbacks ■ Nightmares	■ Beliefs about blame and shame ■ Attitudes to male/female sexuality ■ Low self esteem ■ Control issues – angry or critical towards self and/ or others ■ Unwanted or inappropriate fantasies ■ Compulsions or addictions ■ Suicidal plans
Body	**Emotion**
■ Physical damage from assault ■ Hyper or low arousal ■ Body tension, armouring ■ Pain-fear-tension triangle ■ Disassociation ■ Negative body image ■ Avoidance or indulgence (sexual or food bulimia or anorexia) ■ Somatic illnesses, including sexual and gynaecological issues	■ Overwhelming emotions and feelings ■ Anxieties and fears about safety ■ Terror or panic ■ Depression ■ Self-disgust, shame or humiliation ■ Intimacy and trust issues ■ Anger and communication difficulties ■ Isolation and feeling misunderstood ■ Despair and despondency ■ Suicidal feelings

Figure 19.   The impact of sexual violence.

Studies indicate that male survivors of child sexual abuse might attempt to "prove" their masculinity by having multiple female sexual partners, or they might sexually victimise others and/or engage in dangerous or violent behaviours. Male victims of sexual abuse might develop confusion over their gender and sexual identities; they might have a sense of being inadequate as a man and/or have a sense of having lost power, control, and confidence in their manhood. They might also be left doubting their sexuality, fearing sex, and may have difficulty forming relationships afterwards.

Our cultural and social inconsistencies with regard to sexual violence add to a misunderstanding of the scope and the scale of this phenomenon. This plays a large part in the difficulties in recovery from assaults. We still largely have a notion that sexual assault and childhood sexual abuse offences are committed by strangers, whereas the opposite is true. Most rapists of women are ex-husbands and part-ners, and most abusers of children are people the children know. Perhaps the idea behind our "stranger-danger" thinking allows us to believe that sexual violence is something that happens to other people who were not clever or aware enough to avoid it.

Sexual assault of adults is a traumatic event. When we are in life-threatening or potentially life-threatening situations, our survival circuits come on line. A flood of neurochemicals from the limbic system activates our fight or flight instinct and short-circuits the link to our frontal lobes: we do not register what we think or feel about the situation; the priority is to stay alive. Sometimes, the fight and flight circuits become overwhelmed, leading to disassociation or freezing, like a rabbit in headlights. We can become numb and go on to some sort of automatic pilot. In situations such as rape, going along with something may be a survival attempt, to at least "only" be raped, rather than being raped and mutilated, or raped and murdered. Un-tangling this web can be a very difficult phase for people in recovery.

Humans have to deal with many trials and tribulations throughout our lives, such as tragedy and death. We have a natural capacity to recover from traumas by going through a series of reactions, usually starting with shock. This can take many forms, including disassociation and denial. There will probably be phases of grief, sadness, and anger. The important phase, which becomes complicated in recovery from sexual violence, is the "what if" phase, where we blame ourselves for "allowing" the situation to occur. For example, people say, what if I had walked instead of driving the car on the day of the crash, or what if I hadn't had the argument with my friend or lover the morning before they were killed. Part of recovery is that we work through this phase to realise that had we known beforehand that the traumatic event were going to happen, we probably would have behaved differently.

This is about coming to terms with our powerlessness and the ensuing feelings that this brings, usually more grief and anger. Eventually, we are usually able to find some way of accepting or living with what has happened. This "what if" phase is interrupted for survivors of sexual abuse because, culturally, we do blame them, leading to a much higher incidence of post-trauma stress as people find it difficult to forgive themselves. Work by Herman (1993), Levine (1997), and Rothschild (2000) has contributed hugely to our understanding of post-trauma stress; it has physical and psychological impacts and different levels of trauma. This has also enhanced our knowledge and understanding of the recovery process.

Our legal culture of blame and innocence prefers a much more black-and-white approach, where one person is innocent and the other to blame. This issue, added to our cultural myths and beliefs about sexual violence, is the reason why many people do not want to formally report their assaults. Again, whether to report or not is an individualised need for each survivor. Many feel that reliving the trauma through the courts is too much, many that they will be disbelieved, or they blame themselves anyway. A study in 2003 showed that only twelve per cent of rapes were committed by strangers, and that over two-thirds of cases went no further after being reported to the police. Cases involving intimates were most likely to be discontinued (CER, 2006; Research and Development Statistics Home Office, 2003; Truth about Rape Campaign, 2012). Treatment of survivors by the police themselves has had a bad press in the past, but they now offer a specialist service at The Havens (see www.thehavens.co.uk).

Childhood sexual abuse is an even more complex issue, because a betrayal of trust is most often an additional factor. We now understand about "grooming": how an adult manipulates the child's innocence and relative powerlessness, their physical or emotional needs, to trick them into complying with the adult's demands. Recovery from childhood sexual abuse requires an individualised approach. Not only are there factors such as the duration and extent of the abuse, levels of physical or psychological damage, or who the abuser was in relation to the child, but also consideration needs to be given to the very subjective experience of any of the above.

There are those who engage in consensual sexual violence; this is distinct from sexual abuse, which is not consensual. There has been much discussion about this subject, with some arguing that the pathologising of what is an adult decision to play sexually with BDSM (bondage, dominance, sadomasochism) is an attempt to undermine the liberalisation of sexual attitudes and beliefs that has been long overdue. It is further argued that such attitudes are veiled attempts to pathologise sexual behaviours of sexual minorities, even though many who play with all or any elements of Kink or BDSM are heterosexual. Most BDSM situations are more about playing with power than inflicting pain, and usually involve discussions between those involved about what, where, and how, and include agreements about safe words that mean stop. Kink practices can range from mild to wild. Some people enjoy extreme sports like white water rafting or bungee jumping; some enjoy more extreme forms of sex.

Writers like Morin (1996) and Kort (2003), believe that exploring issues about power, about dominance and submission, can act to heal past wounds of abuse by replaying scenarios but changing elements or endings to more satisfactory ones. Not everyone involved in Kink/ BDSM has a history of sexual violence, but there are some links. It is perhaps a question for the individual about the motivations behind their sexual behaviour and whether this is a problem for them or not. Research by Kahr (2007) into the sexual fantasies of 15,000 people gave us much insight into the range of sexual fantasies people have, but also what might be in their psyches to fuel them. He concluded that although many of the people describing violent or abusive fantasies did not disclose a history of sexual violence *per se*, that further investigation did identify issues that would be perceived as physical and emotional neglect or abuse, within a psychotherapeutic evaluation. The ground-breaking work by Miller (1987, 1991) explored why it is so common for people to "normalise" their childhood experiences and our psychological need to do so. Her later work (2006) describes what she calls "the lingering effects of cruel parenting". Maltz (2010) describes how victims of incest, violence, and sexual abuse may experience compounded feelings of pleasure, pain, and shame while being sexual, and might find it difficult to differentiate fear from sexual excitement.

It is beyond the scope of this book to address recovery from childhood sexual abuse, or sexual violence as an adult, in the depth needed for recovery. However, some excellent books have been written by Bass and Davis (1990), Maltz (1991), Haines (1999), Lew (2004), and Kelly and Maxted (2005), providing programmes to do so. They focus on regaining a sense of integrity of the self, acceptance, and self-care. Herman (1993) suggested the importance of doing recovery work within the context of a safe relationship (with a therapist, within a "survivors" group, or with a trusted friend), because it was within a "relationship" that the abuse occurred. Working through the exercises in this book can help with recovery by helping to re-assert beliefs and values, and gaining a deeper understanding of how our sexual processes work, and how trauma can interrupt our otherwise natural reactions.

As this model is homeodynamic, it is believed that working in any area can also have a positive impact on others. For example, reviewing our beliefs so that we no longer feel self-blame can reduce emotions of anger towards the self, reduce adrenalin in the body, and reduce reactivity in the nervous system and muscle tension. Replacing our most negative thoughts with positive affirmations can create new neural pathways and alter our physiology of stress. This, in turn, allows greater relaxation and more feel-good neurochemicals such as serotonin, which affect our emotional states. Equally, taking greater care of our bodies can make us feel more loving towards ourselves and reduce any critical mind-talk. This can include exercise and good food and sleep habits. Spiritual practices such as meditation can also help calm the mind and the body. A spiritual belief system or philosophical outlook on life can often help us to come to terms with many of the powerless experiences we have as humans by reminding us of our vulnerabilities. Can we strive for the courage to change what we can, the humility to accept what we cannot change, and the wisdom to know the difference? Knowing more explicitly what we like sensually and sexually enables us to make more conscious choices about what type of sexual encounters we want and with whom. Understanding and having compassion for our history and our ensuing reactivity can encourage us to reflect and think before we act, to become more conscious about our sexual behaviour. This, in turn, can make us more confident and trusting about our ability to look after ourselves and, also, more trusting of others.

Exercise   Healing trauma

If you are aware that you have experienced significant trauma in your history, please re-read the exercise "Applying the brakes" at the beginning of the book before you explore this issue more.

Think about one issue that you consider still has an impact in your sexual life now. Do not think about any details of the trauma, but focus instead on the here and now. Think about the circuit of arousal and see if you can identify where it gets interrupted. Explore in turn how you are affected now in your brain, your mind, your body, and your emotions. Are any aspects more affected than others?

If you discover that your brain reflexes are still affected, that you suffer from post traumatic stress symptoms such as flashbacks or nightmares, investigate treatments which might help to alleviate symptoms, such as EMDR (eye movement desensitisation and reprocessing) or "rewind therapy".

If you find that your thoughts, beliefs, and values are still influenced by past events, see if you can identify how you might change them. Explore whether your thinking is based on old or cultural beliefs and evaluate whether they serve you now. Seek out other opinions and beliefs to support any changes you want to make.

If you feel your body is still suffering, consider having some gentle bodywork therapy, such as massage, craniosacral therapy, or Feldenkrais, for example. Ask friends or explore via the Internet until you find a therapy that suits you. You might wish to treat yourself by having sensuous baths with relaxing essential oils, preparing nutritious food for yourself, and making time to rest and relax more.

If you think your emotional life and relationships are still affected, consider some counselling or therapy to work through what impact the trauma may still be having on you. Again, shop around to find the style of therapy that suits you best.

Think about reclaiming your right to sexual pleasure. Go back to the exercises about sensuality and sexual pleasure to remind yourself about the specific things that turn you on. Remember you can use these to switch your arousal circuit back on if you want to.

Evaluate for yourself the achievements you have made in recovering from this trauma already and outline any further challenges you may have. Enlist the help of friends or professionals to support you.

Safer sex

The issue of reproductive and sexual health is the biggest arena where our reproductive model of sex gets us into trouble. We combine sex and reproduction where we need to separate them and we treat them separately where we need to amalgamate them. Our "family planning" clinics, often within a GP practice, provide a variety of contraceptive methods to address reproductive issues, many of which bring other health issues. As discussed earlier, many of our sexual behaviours do not result in reproduction, but can result in sexual health problems. Oral sex, anal sex, or mutual masturbation all become areas for discussion within the different clinical settings, often based in hospitals, that of "sexual health". We have many types of contraception and ways of attempting to control our fertility to allow heterosexual intercourse without risk of pregnancy. Most of these do not protect against sexually transmitted infections (STIs), which are a huge sexual health problem for us now.

Many STIs are asymptomatic, increasing the risk of infecting others. Awareness of a high rate of undiagnosed chlamydial infection led to a national chlamydia screening programme being set up in England in 2003 by the Department of Health, as part of the National Strategy for Sexual Health and HIV. Chlamydia often has no or few symptoms; if untreated, it can lead to serious gynaecological problems, including infertility. Chlamydia is now the most common STI, with new diagnoses increasing from 67,173 in 2000 to 189,612 in 2010. (All data quoted in this section is from the Department of Health online statistics, unless otherwise referenced.) The main STIs of our day are the bacterial infections of syphilis and gonorrhoea, which can be treated with antibiotics, and the viral infections of herpes and genital warts (HPV). Figure 20 shows numbers of new cases diagnosed

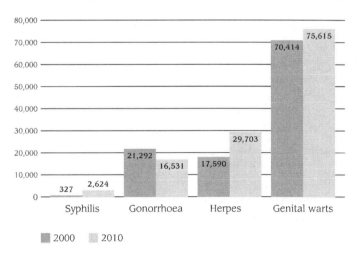

Figure 20. New diagnoses of sexually transmitted infections 2000–2010.

during 2000 and 2010. This shows the huge numbers of viral infections, which bring life-long difficulties. Other viral infections, such as hepatitis, are a major problem, too.

Compared to the HIV awareness campaign in the 1980s, we do not hear much about HIV these days. In 2009, it was reported that there had been a seventeen per cent worldwide reduction in new HIV infections, following the United Nations Declaration of Commitment on HIV/AIDS, signed in 2001. This is particularly so in sub-Saharan Africa and Asia; however, there are signs in some European countries that new HIV infection rates are rising again (World Health Organisation, 2009).

The Terrence Higgins Trust believes that HIV is one of the fastest growing serious health conditions in the UK. Recent statistics taken from the Health Protection Agency (2011) show that

- there are an estimated 86,500 people living with HIV in the UK;
- twenty-six per cent of these people are undiagnosed and do not know about their HIV infection;
- almost 20,000 people with HIV have died of related conditions since the early 1980s;
- there were 6,630 new diagnoses in 2009;
- forty-two per cent of new HIV diagnoses in 2009 were among men who have sex with men.

There are also other conditions not labelled as STIs, including pubic lice, scabies, trichomonaisis, candida, cystitis, and vaginitis, all of which cause sexual health problems for people. The diagnosis of bacterial vaginosis (BV) has become common in the past ten years (about 97,000 cases per year). Recent research has shown links with the viral infection herpes: women with BV are nearly twice as likely to get herpes as women who do not have BV (Hillier, 2008).

So, what are our safer sex strategies, as both national policies and as individuals? Sadly, they show how the confusions between reproductive and sexual health undermine a safer sex ethos. In January 2012, the World Health Organisation is to re-evaluate its contraceptive recommendations, following research in South Africa which has indicated that hormonal contraceptive injections appear to double a woman's risk of contracting HIV and, if she already has HIV, it doubles her risk of transmitting it to her partner compared to women who use no contraception. The reason for the increased risk is not clear, though researchers essentially ruled out the possibility that decreased condom use was a factor (Gastaldo, 2011).

The most common reason cited for using a condom by both men and women in the UK was the prevention of pregnancy, yet less than half cite prevention of infection as well. Around half of men and women in sexual relationships report using condoms, but not always. Of those with multiple partners, less than half always use condoms and twenty-five per cent of women and eighteen per cent of men report never using them. Condom use is much higher in sixteen to twenty-four year olds: seventy per cent of women and eighty-eight per cent of men.

In 2008, mass vaccinations for teenage girls in Britain were planned, using a vaccine (Gardasil) said to "stop cancer" (Moore, 2008): it was to immunise against two strains of HPV (human papilloma virus) that had been identified as precursors to cervical cancer. (There are at least fifteen other strains of HPV, which causes genital warts.) This vaccine was not promoted via health professionals, but gained interest through an emotive campaign aimed at mothers by the drug companies who sell it: "even if it saves only one life, that life might be your daughter's". Much concern was raised that a drug was being marketed to the healthy to protect against a disease that most people will not get, along with worries that it is undermining screening programmes. Research was not carried out on the age group the drugs were to be administered to and Tomljenovic (2011) argues that it presents more health risks than cervical cancer itself. Her research concludes that the clinical trials on Gardasil have been largely inadequate, the efficacy of the vaccine in preventing cervical cancer has not been demonstrated, and that the risks of serious adverse effects are substantial. She believes that the benefits of vaccination have been exaggerated and safety concerns downplayed, thus preventing parents from making informed decisions for their children.

Many believe that the half a billion pounds allocated for this campaign could have been better spent on promoting a much wider safer sex message: that safer sex practices can protect against all sexually transmitted infections and unwanted pregnancies, too. But recent research by the Department of Health in 2009 showed that publicity about STIs had little impact on people, with only thirty-four per cent reporting an increase in condom use. Of those not in a long-term exclusive relationship, fifty-nine per cent said publicity about STIs had no effect on their behaviour (Office for National Statistics, 2011).

Safer sex practices include

- using condoms for vaginal or anal sex;
- using barriers such as dental dams for oral sex;
- good oral hygiene;
- washing and / or using condoms on sex toys;
- taking care to practise safer sex when under the influence of alcohol or other drugs;
- never sharing needles, syringes, or any other injecting equipment.

Condoms are free at sexual health clinics, which are listed on the Internet, in telephone directories, or via NHS Direct (National Aids Trust, 2011).

There are those who always practise safer sex, and those who consider they do not need to, as they are not sexually active or are in an exclusive, monogamous relationship where both partners know they carry no risk. Some people act to protect themselves against pregnancy but not against STIs, and some do neither. So why might this be? There are people who like the thrill of engaging in risky behaviour and others who inadvertently do so while under the influence of alcohol or other drugs. Others seem oblivious to all the risks: a morning after pill may reverse the risk of pregnancy, but not of catching an STI.

We rarely see safer sex being practised or referred to during "lovemaking scenes" on television, in films, or in pornography. It is as if we prefer not to see ourselves consciously choosing to be sexual. Do we prefer to think (and want) to just get so carried away that we do not think about consequences until later? This may be part of our romantic view of sex, or our belief that the sex urge is so strong nothing can (or should) get in its way. It could also be an indicator of the degree of shame we feel still about owning and honouring our sexual desires. Coming out of shame would necessitate witnessing our desire, admitting in advance that we might well behave sexually, and being prepared to practise safer sex. We do not have to "stop" to put on a condom; doing so can be part of sex play. It depends on your attitude. Some think others will not like you being prepared, that it is presumptuous for a man or slutty for a woman, neither of which are true.

Acknowledging your desire and wanting to have safe fun respects yourself and others, and indicates sexual self-esteem.

Within a model of psychosexual health, safer sex is not just about the avoidance of STIs and pregnancy, but about emotional and physical safety, too. It includes drug and alcohol awareness, and how they may undermine safer sex practices or link with risky behaviour. Attention is given to self-care, choices, and assertiveness, not just knowing for ourselves what we want and desire, but communicating and negotiating this with others. For example, we could teach our girls how to interpret the clear signs of their brief monthly fertile phase; they (and a partner) could then make decisions about which sexual activities they may want to engage in at different stages of her fertility cycle. This would need a cultural shift in attitudes that have been discussed in this book; it would require coming out of shame.

Exercise   Sexual health workout

Think about your sexual health in same way you might consider your physical health if you were to consider getting more healthy. If you were to review your physical health, you might address your diet, what exercise you get, your sleeping habits, and your stress levels, for example.

For your sexual health review, you may want to consider having a check-up at a sexual health clinic. You will find details of your nearest clinic via the Internet or at your local health centre or hospital.

Do you consider that your current sexual beliefs and values are healthy? Do you consider that your current sexual practices are healthy? Do you practise safer sex? Do you use alcohol or recreational drugs as part of your sexual life? Do some of your practices involve risk or harm to yourself or others?

What impact do you think any of the above have on your body or your mental or emotional well-being? Write about what you think and feel about your answers to these questions. Identify any changes you would like to make and consider how you may do so.

Relationships

We have many types of relationships: with family, friends, colleagues, and neighbours. They vary in the time and the importance that we give to them. We also have many types of sexual relationships. Some people choose committed long-term relationships with one person, others prefer one-off or casual sexual encounters with different people, and others a combination of these at different times of their life. During a lifetime, many adults will go through stages of wishing to create the types of sexual relationships they want, and encountering difficulties or frustrations with this. Some might be in a state of heartache through being unable to have a relationship with someone they desire, for a variety of reasons, or through being rejected. Others might have lost loved ones through break-up, divorce, or bereavement. There are those trying to maintain and sustain long-term relationships, dealing with difficult life stages, conflict, or loss of desire. We think and talk about our sexual relationships a lot, often involving much disappointment, confusion, and grief. They preoccupy much of our time and energy. Sexual relationships can also bring great pleasure and joy and fulfil our desires for bonding, allowing us to love and feel loved. They can allow us to relax and to fulfil all the socialising circuits of the brain (caring, curiosity, play, and physical contact).

For those seeking a relationship, it can sometimes seem like a merry dance around how to meet someone, let alone finding the sort of person you want to meet. The Internet or speed-dating might seem to offer easier opportunities but can also demand a high degree of confidence and self-esteem. For many, the whole topic can feel like an emotional rollercoaster that is difficult to navigate. There is a need to believe that "someone special" is out there and feel trust about the potential of meeting them. There is a stage of meeting people, getting excited, and hoping it will work out between you. Sometimes it does, or might do for a while, but then flounders. Then there may be disappointment and all the ensuing feelings, or a worry that you are not good enough. Eventually, people regain their confidence to go out and try again, and again and again. Many question their expectations: am I asking too much, should I settle for less? Sometimes they may despair that they might never meet someone.

Cross-cultural and same sex couples can encounter added difficulties even once they do meet someone. They might have acted outside of the perceived norm or expectation of their culture of origin, which can be experienced through national identity, race, colour, ethnicity, religion, class, education, or sexual orientation. They might have experienced racism, oppression, discrimination, or prejudice from family of origin, wider community, and society, both as individuals, and as a couple. They may need to negotiate issues regarding parenting, sexual beliefs, attitudes and behaviours, gender roles and traditions, and expression of emotion and conflict management. It should be noted that not all cultural differences cause difficulty or distress in a couple, and that not all problems intercultural couples encounter are culturally based.

Same sex couples might need to deal with homophobia and lack of acceptance by their families of origin, local communities, and the wider society. There could be different attitudes and behaviours in "coming out", in sexual attitudes and behaviours, and issues regarding parenting and reproduction. They have different legal issues to contend with. Some find that a lack of role models and traditional and social rituals to support couples can add to stresses of being in a relationship.

Throughout this book, we have been exploring a relationship with our own sexuality. Some analysis of the psychology of relationships can help to raise awareness of our unconscious (reactive) desires and attractions. This, in turn, allows us to become more conscious and think (reflect) about what type of sexual relationships we want, and with what type of person. Work in psychotherapy and neuroscience shows that humans are hardwired for relationships and connections. As discussed earlier, an infant is dependent on the attachment relationship with its primary carer to develop its brain functioning; its ability to soothe and manage its feelings are so vital for mental health and emotional well-being. Many believe our early attachment patterns inform our unconscious choices of relationships as adults.

Kaufman and Raphael (1996) say we have a predominant affect (developed through our childhood experiences) which leads to patterns in adult relationships. For example, when enjoyment is our predominant mode, our relationship pattern will be for continuity and commitment, and excitement leads to desires for novelty and new lovers. When fear and excitement are linked we are likely to pursue danger, and when fear and shame are linked, we are more likely to abandon relationships. They believe that shame as a primary affect leads to hiding, avoidance, and entering abusive relationships, and contempt leads to distancing others, superiority, and creating abusive relationships.

Goldhor Lerner (1990) describes intimacy as a dance: that we need to be two separate beings, which are able to tolerate our differences and can trust that we will not be abandoned when we are in the place of separation. We need to be able to move together to make contact, and, at times, merge. In this place, we need to trust that in time we will separate and not become engulfed by the other. As a couple dance their intimacy, they move in and out and in-between these three places, feeling comfortable (enough) in all (Figure 21). And clearly, this is not always easy.

Hendrix (1993) believes that we select a mate who has the potential to help us heal our childhood wounds and become a more whole, loving person. This selection is based on three things:

1.   They have our primary care-givers' *positive and negative* traits.
2.   These traits may represent our lost self, parts of us that were unacceptable to our care-givers and were therefore abandoned by us
3.   They may also embody our disowned traits—aspects of ourselves we never developed and so want another to embody for us.

He says that after the falling in love stage, there *inevitably* follows a power struggle stage, because we have entered this relationship with the unconscious expectation that our partner will love us in the way our parents never did. He believes our aim is to work with, not against, the unconscious purpose of the relationship, an opportunity to heal our intimacy wounds by creating an alliance to help each other become more assertive and less defensive by learning about and embracing our own dark side to avoid projecting it on to our partners and to develop hidden facets within ourselves. Rather than seeing our partner as "the problem", we are offered the challenge to address our own difficulties with intimacy. There have been some excellent books written to suggest ways for couples to work with their difficulties, including Geraghty (2003), Green and Flemons (2004), and Martin-Sperry (2004).

Separation	Contact	Merger
① ②	① ②	①②

Figure 21.   The dance of intimacy.

Given the childhood wounds most of us have, love does not come easy. This is not about "blaming the parents", as their parenting skills will have been handed down to them. Perhaps this is a time in history where our basic needs (for food and shelter) are most often met; we have the luxury of considering the emotional qualities of our lives. We have the knowledge now of our childhood needs to develop into personally and socially mature adults. But, for the moment, we still have much to learn about love. O'Dwyer (2011) discusses work by Fromm, in which he argues that love is an art which must be developed and practised with commitment and humility; it requires knowledge, courage, and effort. He says it requires the practice of four essential elements:

- care: concern for welfare, commitment of time and effort;
- responsibility: willingness to respond to physical and psychological needs;
- respect: the need for differentiation—ability to experience love is based on the individual's commitment to the freedom and autonomy of both partners;
- knowledge: of the other, not my perspectives or concerns.

O'Dwyer says "milk" is the basic care and affirmations that we all need and she adds a fifth essential element, which she calls "honey": the sweetness of life, the happiness in being alive and having a sense of enjoyment in the very existence of the other.

Bader and Pearson (1998) have outlined a developmental model of adult relationships based on Mahler's child development model (see Figure 22, first column, in bold), which also fits with the stages in Hendrix's psychosocial model (see Figure 22, first column, in upper case). Figure 22 shows the stages and the challenges we face.

Lack of sexual desire and managing conflict within a relationship are the two main difficulties that present in couple work, and they are linked. Both are about our fire energy, our passion, how we experience it and how we express it. Some find themselves creative, spontaneous, and want to use their passion to make something wonderful and joyous. Others struggle with this aspect of themselves. Their creativity and free expression of their passions might have been quashed in childhood. They might have been discouraged to "be" themselves or have grown up around arguing, fighting, and conflict.

HENDRIX Mahler	Adult Relationships	Challenges
ATTACHMENT **Symbiotic** Fusion with the primary care giver	"Being madly in love", merging, intense bonding, forming attachment. Nurturing freely given and received	To build a strong attachment foundation
EXPLORATION **Separation/** **individuation** More alertness to the environment	If attachment foundation strong, couple able to move to differentiation	If not successful in building strong foundation may get stuck in Symbiosis as **Enmeshment** – avoid conflict and minimize difference or **Hostile Dependent** – stuck in anger and conflict
IDENTITY **Differentiation** Increasing sense of self and other. *Learning of physical* *boundaries*	Re-establish boundaries, more aware of differences as well as similarities. This is challenging and exciting	If couple have not successfully negotiated Symbiosis, this may bring disillusionment
COMPETENCE **Practicing** Energy is directed outwards, *differentiation is* *occurring well*	Individuals engaging outside of the relationship; possible decrease in empathy and increase in self- centeredness	Issues of self-esteem, individual power and worthiness come to the fore. Conflicts may intensify, requiring good problem solving skills
CONCERN **Rapprochement** Time of independence and regression. *Power* *struggles*	Well defined individual identities allows for more intimacy and emotional nurturance	Vulnerabilities re-emerge; alternating times of intimacy and independence. Less fear of 'engulfment'; more trust in a strong self of 'us'
INTIMACY **Consolidation** Constancy *Internalised sense* *of care giver*	Mutual interdependence A relationship based on a foundation of growth rather than need	

Figure 22.   Bader and Pearson's developmental model of relationships.

Healthy differentiation is vital to keep passion alive in relationships, and so are good communication skills. The more you know yourself, the more you empathise with an "other"; the more clearly you communicate your needs with appropriate assertiveness, the more you are willing to negotiate and use co-operative power, the happier your relationships will be. An important issue regarding resolving conflict in relationships is to pay attention to the language we use in communication. When we make "I" statements, such as "I think" or "I feel", rather than "we", "one", or "you", we take ownership of our comments and make it clear that we are talking about ourselves rather than other people. Making distinctions about what we do not want to do rather than what we are unable to or cannot do also helps to clarify a situation, as does using the word "could" when appropriate, rather than "should". Using generalisations such as "you always" or "you never" are often experienced as merely criticism. Whereas being specific gives information and direction about what could be changed. For example: when you did (whatever it was), I felt (whatever you felt) and I would prefer it if in future you would . . . (make suggestions).

The Conflict Resolution Network (2012) has devised some guidelines for fair fighting, listed below.

- *Do I want to resolve the conflict?*—Be willing to fix the problem.
- *Can I see the whole picture, not just my own point of view?*—Broaden your outlook.
- *What are the needs and anxieties of everyone involved?*—Write them down.
- *How can we make this fair?*—Negotiate.
- *What are the possibilities?*—Think up as many solutions as you can. Pick the one that gives everyone more of what they want.
- *Can we work it out together?*—Treat each other as equals.
- *What am I feeling? Am I too emotional?*—Could I get more facts, take time out to calm down, tell them how I feel?
- *What do I want to change?*—Be clear. Attack the problem, not the person.
- *What opportunity can this bring?*—Work on the positives, not the negatives.
- *What is it like to be in their shoes?*—Do they know I understand them?

- *Do we need a neutral third person?*—Could this help us to understand each other and create our own solutions?
- *How can we both win?*—Work towards solutions where everyone's needs are respected.

Bedroom politics include issues of power. Historically, a man had a right to sex from his wife; rape within marriage became a crime in Britain in 1994. In many countries and cultures, a patriarchal view of marriage still exists. For many trying to develop a more egalitarian way of being in long-term relationships, with regard to housework and child-rearing for example, they are not sure how this equates with their sexual life. We need a degree of conflict, of frisson within a relationship for it to stay passionate. There needs to be a sense of other, of difference, for there to be attraction, to create a spark. Perel (2007) says we may confuse merger with love, which is a bad omen for sex. In her view, love needs the two pillars of surrender and autonomy, and eroticism thrives in the space between the self and the other. Sex is an arena where we can leave aside our cultural niceties and get on with being our raw, spontaneous selves, and follow our desires in the moment. Perel believes that the interest displayed in Kink/BDSM often has far less to do with pain or wanting to hurt than with wanting to play with power. She sees this as a subversion of cultural abuses of power, where those in authority dictate to those they wield power over. In bondage and dominance play, people can dialogue and agree exactly what, how, and for how long. Many people experience a sense of powerlessness in their lives at times, so to be able to play sexually with having power can feel fun and liberating. Equally, many have demanding jobs or lives caring for others, so that surrendering, letting someone else make all the decisions, can feel a relief and be relaxing. Schnarch (1998, 2002) also believes it is not a lack of closeness which might undermine a couple's sex life, but too much. His work on resurrecting sex and the place of passion in long-term relationships includes a relationship with your own sexuality primarily, your own desires and preferences. Also an ability to accept the differences in a partner, and both being willing to talk, to tussle, to negotiate, or dominate or surrender, at different times on that edge and in the space in-between. He suggests a range of ways to reignite passion in relationships that are faltering. Love and Robinson (1995) also discuss the desire that many people have for passionate intimate lovemaking within a long-term relationship. Their work provides a sexual style survey which individuals complete and map, then share with their partner to identify areas of strength and issues of challenge. They also suggest ways of overcoming difficulties. Many exercises in this book will have helped your self-awareness; you might want to choose some to do with a partner, either together or separately, and then compare.

Exercise   Your relationships

Explore your patterns in relationships. How do you relate to yourself: do you feel connected to your body and your emotions; is your internal dialogue kind or critical?

Think about how you are in relationships with family, friends, and colleagues. Do you generally find them easy or difficult? Do you find it easy to negotiate and get your needs met, or are you often left feeling disappointed? Do you find them easy to navigate or conflictual, frustrating? Is it easier with people you are very close with or with people you know less well? Can you see a pattern in how you relate? Is it similar to how you relate to yourself?

Now think about your sexual relationships. How are they similar or different to the patterns outlined above? Identify one thing you would like to change in how you relate and consider how you could do that.

Soul food

We have reviewed many topics in this book with regard to sexuality. Through the exercises, you have been invited to an in-depth exploration about your beliefs and where they came from, presenting an opportunity for review and reflection. This has, I hope, brought more clarity to your thinking about your preferences and tastes, allowing you to know more about your sexual values and what is really important to you. Providing intricate details about our body's sexual functioning has clarified the distinctions between reproductive processes and the potential for sexual pleasure that we have. This allows our thinking to move away from sexual intercourse as "real sex", which minimises the intrinsic value of "foreplay", and encourages us to value all the sexual behaviours we might want to express. The exercises offer a chance to explore your own unique body, to become intimate with yourself, and discover your own sensual and sexual pleasure.

Understanding the neurochemistry of sexual functioning and the role of our unique histories in our sexual desires help us to make more sense of our reactivity, providing us with more choice about our behaviour. We have learnt more also about the impact of our childhoods on our brain patterning and, therefore, our expectations of the "other". This again shows our human need for attachment and relationship: how we instinctually move towards what gives us pleasure and away from what does not, and how this gets confused when our childhood needs are not met. Exploring the relationship between our thinking mind, our reactive brain, and our body leads us into the world of emotions, of energy in motion in the body, where the interrelatedness between the internal aspects of ourselves becomes more evident. Our human interrelatedness also becomes more evident, as well as the role of emotions and basic human brain circuits in ways of relating to each other. The exercises encourage emotional intelligence in how we relate to ourselves and to others and allow us to familiarise ourselves with energy charges in the body, first with emotions and then with our sexual energy.

This exploration of self then turns towards the other, to social and cultural issues to explore some shadow issues such as sexual shame and sexual violence, the impact of which is heart-breaking. This book is an attempt to counter cultural shame by offering factual information, within a cultural context, and promote a celebration of our sexual capacities. It explores stages in our psychosocial development and our relational needs to see how this may correlate with our developing sexuality. The idea of us being sexual people, and the wide range of ways of expressing ourselves sexually, is emphasised throughout, rather than the notion of sex as an act. Expanding on the notion of feelings as an interaction between our reactivity, somatic experiences, emotions, and thoughts allows us to make more conscious choices and to see the elements involved in sexual self-esteem.

We have a variety of views, tastes, and preferences around our sexuality. A further aim of this book is for us to think about and evaluate our social and cultural relationship with sexuality, and consider what we are teaching our children, discussing in the media, and viewing on the Internet. This free, amazing gift for fun and pleasure does not get the good press it should; we do not celebrate our sexual potential. In the West, we are encouraged to want *things* rather than relationships, to have attachments to and value objects (cars, phones, etc.), rather than to people. We have developed an objectified relationship to our sexuality. Our bodies, rather than being honoured as a free source of sensual and sexual pleasure, are offered up to be pruned and plucked, shaved and cut, to be altered into a mono-cultured image of beauty. We are offered thousands of potentially not-healthy products to glamorise us and are exposed to thousands of sexualised images to sell us *things*. We are encouraged to overcome our cultural shame about sexuality by being shameless, by objectifying ourselves and others.

Although many religions seek to diminish the pleasure principle, thoughts and beliefs about "sacred sexuality" take a very different approach where the role of sexual pleasure is seen as vital, as a joyous aspect to being human. The quality of sexual expression is seen as essential, where intimacy and conscious connectedness are at the heart and relationships valued and respected. Carrellas (2007) discusses concepts like bliss and ecstasy and how they differ from the adrenalised states we are encouraged to confuse them with. Adrenalin is part of the biochemical mix of sexual arousal, but it also creates a release of cortisol, which takes us into survival patterns and has longer term deleterious effects on our bodies, including clouding our thinking and slowing down our digestive system. She suggests that the simple path to ecstasy includes continually staying in the present moment, not trying too hard, dropping expectations and judgements, and learning to be more conscious in sexual encounters, while surrendering to being in the present moment.

Many Eastern traditions and complementary medicine systems are aware of the energy systems of the body, including the meridians used in acupuncture and the electromagnetic fields utilised in kinesiology. One system is that of the chakras: that we have an energetic life force which spirals up the body through seven centres. Some can see or perceive this energy; we can all experience it through intention and guided visualisation. Sexual energy can be raised through doing this alongside conscious breathing techniques. The starting place to focus attention is the first or "base" chakra, which is located on the perineum between the anus and the genitals, related to grounding and survival. The focus then moves up to the second chakra, in the belly, the centre of relationships, sexuality, and creativity, then up to the solar plexus, the place of will, of self-esteem, courage, and trust. The intention can be to focus on breathing and imagining drawing the energy up from the genitals through the energy centres. The next chakra is the heart, the centre of compassion and love; and the next, the throat chakra, the place for communication, creative expression, and choice. The sixth chakra, called the third eye, is located at the forehead between the eyebrows, and is seen as the centre for intuition and wisdom. The crown chakra, at the top of the head, is related to bliss, higher love, and a connection to spirituality. Taking time to pay attention to breathing, to draw the sexual energy up through these energy centres can invigorate the body and result in orgasms that are experienced through the whole body rather than just focused in the genital area.

In mainstream culture, talk of tantric sex is somewhat ridiculed and laughed off as some sort of weird gymnastics. Lightwoman (2004) explains Tantra as an embodied experience, being truly present to your somatic body and breath awareness, and learning to ride waves of energy. A tantric encounter might start with "eye gazing", two people spending some time just looking at each other, seeing and being seen by each other, a crucial element to coming out of shame. This is about consciously experiencing touching another's body and being touched, kissing and being kissed, deeply experiencing being in a sexual encounter and the impact this is having on your body, mind, and heart.

The heart is very connected to sexuality, as the heart and the genitals both have smooth muscle, which responds differently to other muscles in the body. Buhner (2004) explains how the heart can be seen as so much more than a pump for our circulatory system: it is also an endocrine gland, making and releasing numerous hormones, a generator of electromagnetic messages, and a part of the central nervous system, with direct links to the limbic system. He goes further, to describe how the heart is an organ of perception and communication. The heart is also our metaphorical place of love, and, for many sharing sexual expression in the context of love, is where the delights of passion can be experienced as the most exquisite. This is not to imply that such experiences can only happen in committed long-term relationships; this is about a relationship with the self. Being conscious and present can bring sexual delights through self-pleasuring or in an encounter with someone you have met for the first time.

We know we have needs for sex just as we have for food. In recent years, we have changed our cultural attitudes to food; we are becoming much more aware of what foods are healthy, and what are not. We know we need proteins, complex carbohydrates, vitamins, and

minerals. We know that processed foods are often stripped of ingredients needed for good digestion, and that junk foods are high in satu-
rated fats, salt, and sugar, with all the associated health implications.
We have become more aware of our nutritional needs, both for our
physical and emotional well-being.

So, what if we were to consider the same for our sexual needs;
what would be the equivalence? Within the homeodynamic model,
we know we have attraction to others triggered from our back brain,
informed by our history and memories. Our thinking, beliefs, and
choices are bound also by our unique social and cultural experiences.
How we experience our bodies and our emotions is also affected by
a culture that mainly denies the value of either. How do we turn
this around and begin to think about what is nutritious for us sexually?

Moran (2011) gives a good example where she describes the difference between lap-dancing and strip clubs as opposed to burlesque,
where artistes of the latter (with a range of body sizes and shapes)
may also sing, talk, and laugh *with* their audience while they dance
and creatively explore their female-centred sexuality. It perhaps
reflects the difference between factory farming and the free-range
production of food.

Many of the exercises in this book have encouraged you to explore
what sexual nutrients you want and value, and also to evaluate what
of your thinking and behaviour is nutritious, in that it satiates your
body, mind, and soul. Does your sexual diet leave you feeling good,
in a state of physical, psychological, and emotional well-being? It is
not to say certain beliefs or behaviours are in themselves not nutritious, but more, for the moment, to include an integrative appraisal.
A vegetarian might agree that meat can be a wholesome source of
protein, but would still not want it as part of their diet, and may even
campaign around the politics of meat. To create a sexually nutritious
diet, we need to individualise our needs physically, emotionally, and
spiritually, whatever that might mean. The context here is about
beliefs and values, what satisfies your heart and soul. To have
contemplated the range of "sexual foods" available and balance your
ingestion of them, in line with your emotional needs and belief
systems, will allow for the best digestion and absorption, invigorating
your body, mind, and heart. This, in turn, can lead to a good sense of
sexual self-esteem.

Exercise   Sexual diet

Write down the first four things that you believe about sex and sexuality that come to mind. Reflect on what you have written and consider if you think they are nutritious for you or not. Think about why you think what you do.

Now write down your four most common sexual behaviours. Again, reflect on what you have written and consider if you think they are nutritious for you or not. Be specific about why you think what you do: is it what the behaviours are, or how you engage in them? Does your body feel depleted afterwards, or invigorated and satiated? How do you feel after, proud or ashamed?

Now consider your emotional needs and how your history has made you who you are. In this context, how do you evaluate your beliefs and behaviours? What is it like to consider your sexual diet in the context of your desires, your beliefs, and your physical and emotional needs?

Write down four things you would like to change in each of these areas and consider how you could do that.

Make love, not war

In the homeodynamic model for sexuality, we have separated the different aspects of mind, body, brain, and emotion, although they are interrelational because they are all constantly affected by, and affect, each other. The individual has been discussed within a social and cultural context, integrating thinking from multi-disciplinary fields. This is just a model, a way of thinking about these different elements to try to understand better what may be the ingredients for a healthy sexual self-esteem. Please feel free to use this as you wish and to discard anything that does not work for you. There might be other elements you wish to add or topics that have not been included that are of interest to you. There are many resources, some included here and others in books or on the Internet, for you to explore further.

The Mind section explored our beliefs and sexual values and how they have been influenced by religion, shame, and a cultural exploitation of sexuality, as well as what we learnt as children. The Body section described our sexual functioning, including how the vulva, not the vagina, is women's primary sexual organ. The role of the nervous system, endocrine system, and respiratory system in the sexual arousal process was also explained. The Brain section explored our passion, urges, and sexual desire. It outlined the role of neurochemicals in sexual functioning, and described the difference between the survival and the socialising brain circuits: the former activating the adrenal system and the latter, activating "feel good" substances instead. How childhood experiences have an impact on our reflexive reactions was discussed, and how we can use our thinking capabilities to make choices about how we behave. The section on Emotion explored emotional intelligence and outlined the impacts of trauma on our bodies and hearts. We discussed safer sex as not just avoiding pregnancy or infection, but including our physical and emotional safety as well.

We do not have a good relationship with our sexuality culturally. We do not seem to be at peace with this aspect of humanity, and we certainly do not celebrate it. In fact, there are many ways in which we seem to be at war, either through the constraints of cultural shame or the shamelessness of our modern times. The main attack is on our bodies. Ultra-thin women are valued as icons of beauty and cosmetic surgery (which used to be called plastic surgery) is now normalised. Most of us have our email spam boxes filled daily with adverts for penis enlargement products. Much focus is on looking sexy rather than feeling sexy, on being thin rather than feeling good about being a healthy body mass index (the ratio between our weight, height, and body frame). Many "health and beauty products" contain questionable chemicals which deserve further research to ascertain their safety, given the health concerns of their impacts on cancers, hormonal disruption, and other reproductive health issues. For many years, sex has been used to sell things; there are now hundreds of things we can buy to "make us sexy".

Sexual violence is another way that war is waged against our sexuality, both in that it happens and in our cultural treatment of victims. Almost as if it is a cultural blind spot, we teach our children about "stranger-danger" and routinely dismiss rape crimes when the attacker is someone known to the victim, when, in fact, the majority of perpetrators are not strangers. These cultural mythologies distort the reality and extent of sexual violence in our society. This, in turn, makes recovery from such trauma more complex and difficult.

Another assault is how our need for the erotic has become hijacked by an industry that just wants to profit from us regardless of the quality or value of what is being sold. Its main aim is to entice new customers and offer novelty to its existing customers. One example of this is the recent development of what is called pseudo child pornography (Dines, 2010). In 2002, lobbying from the pornography industry resulted in a redefining of the 1996 Child Pornography Prevention Act in America. Whereas it was illegal to have visual depictions that appear to be a minor engaging in sexually explicit conduct, the ruling was changed so that the performers were not allowed actually to be aged under eighteen, regardless of appearance. This led to a proliferation of "teen porn" or "teen sex" sites (nine million sites). Here, women appear in childlike clothes, school uniforms, no make-up, holding teddy bears. In complete contrast to the derogatory language used in "adult" porn, the language used here towards the women is "sweetie", "cutie", and body parts are described as "petite" or "tight". The story often involves an older man, such as a schoolteacher or sports instructor, using affection, caressing, and kissing to cajole the "girl" from her innocence to find her eagerness to lose her virginity.

How can we reclaim our sexuality from consumerism to develop a sexual self-esteem where it is valued, respected, honoured, and celebrated as a great gift? When some people began to question the nutritional value of junk food being sold to us via fast food stores, and microwavable food, we did not see them as "anti-food"—if anything, the opposite. The allure for quickly available, cheap food is obvious; it was good quality, healthy food that was being called for. Nigel Slater's *Real Fast Food* (1993) is an example of a more creative solution. To demand healthy sexualised goods as consumers, we need to overcome our cultural shame. We need to feel comfortable to be consciously sexual, to see ourselves and to allow ourselves to be seen by others. We need sex affirmative resources that encourage us to feel proud of our sexual arousal and pleasure, to freely play with our fire energy. We need resources to spark our own imaginations and creativity.

The macro-historian Riane Eisler says humans create two types of societies. One is "dominator cultures", like ours, where hierarchical models of power persist, along with beliefs that humans are essentially violent, selfish, and greedy and that suffering is the "human condition". The other is "partnership cultures", with more power sharing and collective responsibility, where social structures are created to support life as an essentially joyful and connected experience. A society like ours invites a cynicism about the possibility of change, of us becoming less abusive and more honouring and respectful of many things, including our sexuality (Banks, 2011). Our economic model of relentlessly pursuing growth, until the inevitable bust and depressions, is similar to the eating disorder, bulimia. Our consumer society encourages an addiction model where we should always want more, so we never feel satiated. The social costs include rising rates of stress, and emotional and physical ill-health.

Gerhardt (2010) says that society can be seen as the mega family, where social values are passed on at an unconscious level. She says most people lack the emotional security that really matters, so they seek attachment to material goods.

Secure emotional attachments as children are developed through the experience of relationships in which we can learn to self-regulate, to co-operate, and develop empathy. It is through touch and human connection that serotonin and dopamine pathways are nourished, which then reduce stress through the production of oxytocin. Our sexualised behaviour, which relies on adrenalin, activates the survival circuits, with detrimental consequences to our health. Those that are relational trigger the socialising circuits instead. Intimacy can be spelt out as "In-to-me-see". As discussed earlier, being seen and accepted by an "other" is an important aspect of coming out of shame. Relatedness can be seen as the bridge between our existential need for uniqueness and our desires for connection. It is a two-way flow between giving and receiving, and between strength and vulnerability. It is this relational aspect of our sexuality that we need to address.

Brown (2010) conducted some research into why some people are happier than others, having a good sense of self-worth, while others do not. She believes it is shame that undermines our sense of self-esteem. To feel a good sense of self-esteem, we need to feel worthy of being loved, feel accepted and acceptable to be in connection, and feel a right to belong. In order to find this, we need to be willing and able to show our vulnerabilities, to allow ourselves to be imperfect, and be allowed to learn from the mistakes we might make. She says we need courage and compassion to overcome our fears about not being good enough, that we should strive for authenticity and uniqueness, and welcome this in others. Empathy is crucial for good social relationships, whereas anonymity makes it easier for us to exploit. Aims for perfectionism move us back into shame and low self-worth. Macy and Young Brown (1998) explain "holonic systems" (similar to the homeodynamic model), which honour the uniqueness and importance of each different part of the whole. The system self generates from spontaneously adaptive co-operation between the parts, in benefit of the whole. We need a diversity of organs, cells, neurochemicals, etc., to be just what they are and to do their job, and to be in a feedback loop with other parts of the system. For example, it would not be good if the heart tried to become a lung, as each is equally important. For a healthy sexual society, we need a diversity of tastes, preferences, and sexual orientations, too.

If we were sex affirmative as individuals and as a culture, we could see sexual pleasure as a soothing, rejuvenating, ecstatic, free way to counterbalance the pains and struggles of human existence. We need to reclaim the pleasure principle: that we have as much right to fun and play as the demands put on us to work. We have a right to leisure and to enjoy our lives, too. We can do this by making our own sexual stories, fine-tuned to our own desires and specific tastes and preferences, based on our knowledge of ourselves. This conscious celebration is needed to bring us out of shame, to reclaim our family jewels as a precious, life-enhancing, free, creative energy. I hope the tide is turning about our attitudes to sex and sexuality. It would be wonderful for us to break out of our cultural shame, to stop focusing on sex as something we do, to honour our relational needs, and develop an ease about being emotional, sensual, and sexual beings. Banks (2011), in her work with the Transition movement, explores how to address denial of our needs to change. She says the scale of the problem can leave us feeling overwhelmed, so that we shut down as a survival mechanism in the face of this "trauma". We need to engage socially, to share our thoughts and feelings, so as to not feel alone or isolated. This recovery process allows us to move through to empowerment, with an ability to take action again. In a similar way to overcoming sexual shame, we need to name what is being lost, to acknowledge the scale of the problem, feel and move through the pain and grief, to enable healing to occur.

Figure 23 considers the homeodynamic model in alignment with the elements of fire, air, earth, and water, used within many spiritual traditions, and asks, what is at the heart? If we consider all the elements of our sexuality, what is the synergy created when we bring them altogether? It is suggested that psychosexual health means people feeling good about what they think and feel about sex, as well as how they behave. Good sexual self- esteem flows from acting in ways that leaves a person feeling proud, knowing that their sexual life is enhancing their physical, mental, and emotional well-being. We

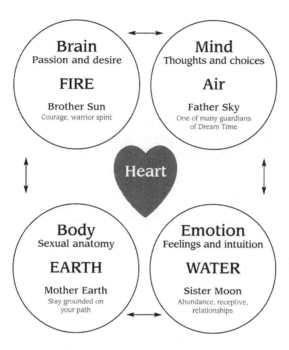

Figure 23.   An elemental homeodynamic model.

have seen that our sexual drive is so much more than a reproductive urge. It is more than a biological urge as well, because, although we can and do self-pleasure, our desire often includes wanting to be sexual with someone else, that we want to connect and be relational, we want to kiss and touch, and to be kissed and touched by another.

Making love triggers the release of feel-good chemicals such as oxytocin, dopamine, and serotonin. It allows us to play, gives us pleasure, and relieves pain. It is good for our physical, mental, and emotional health. Intimate, respectful, and loving relationships are good for us, both our relationship with ourselves and those we have with others. We can have fast sex or slow sex; we can have wonderful love-making alone or with someone we have just met. We can be a gourmet cook and still sometimes just want a snack. Our tastes and preferences may vary. It is not a hierarchy of what is best; it is a circular view of sex. *LoveSex* has provided an opportunity for you to re-evaluate your sexuality. I hope you now feel more empowered to create a nutritious sexual diet that suits your preferences and tastes, that you can love and honour your sexuality, that you can love sex and respect those you share your body with. I hope you can have a sexual life that you feel proud of, which leaves you with a good sense of sexual self-esteem.

Exercise   Review of Part IV

Read back through the exercises for this section and what you have written in your journal. Take some time to reflect on your exploration and to evaluate your work. Which exercises did you like and which ones did you not like? Think about why.

What have you discovered about yourself emotionally, and how comfortable you are with your feelings?

What have you discovered about your relationship to shame; does it have an impact on you and if so, how? Think about what changes you could make to feel more proud instead.

What have you discovered about your relationship to sexual play? Do you have as much fun as you would like to?

If you have been hurt around your sexuality, are there any ways in which you continue to re-enact that hurt? Can you identify any things you could do to help to heal yourself?

What have you discovered about yourself in relationships? Do you have the relationships you would like? If not what are the things that get in the way? Is there anything you want to change? If so, how could you do that?

What is your relationship to your sexuality: is it kind and loving, are you good friends?

Are there any exercises that you would like to do again? If so, notice what is similar or different if you do them a second time.

Read your reviews from each of the other sections as well. Write some things for yourself about your sexual preferences and tastes. Remind yourself about what turns you on, and what turns you off, sensually and sexually. Consider your sexual beliefs, along with the sexual behaviours that you value for yourself. Decide what type of sexual relationships you want to have and what would be a satiating, nutritious sexual diet for you.

Talk to someone, write or draw something about how you are thinking and feeling having done this work.

FURTHER READING

Anand, M. (1990). *The Art of Sexual Ecstasy.* London: Aquarian Press.

Anderson, B. (2002). *Tantra for Gay Men.* Los Angeles, CA: Alyson Books.

Chopra, D. (1989). *Quantum Healing.* New York: Bantam.

Crowe, M., & Ridley, J. (2002). *Therapy with Couples.* Oxford: Blackwell Science.

Cox, T. (1999). *Hot Sex.* London: Corgi.

Cox, T. (1999). *Hot Relationships.* London: Corgi.

Deida, D. (1997). *It's a Guy Thing.* Deerfield Beach, FL: Health Communications.

Dethlefsen, T., & Dahlke, R. (1990). *The Healing Power of Illness.* Shaftesbury: Element Books.

Ensler, E. (2001). *The Vagina Monologues.* London: Virago.

Goldstone, S. (1999). *The Ins and Outs of Gay Sex.* New York: Dell.

Hite, S. (2007). *Oedipus Revisited.* Mount Pleasant, SC: Arcadia Books.

Hunter, M. (1991). *Abused Boys.* New York: Random House.

Jeffreys, S. (2005). *Beauty and Misogyny: Harmful Cultural Practices in the West.* Hove: Routledge.

Kass-Annese, B., & Danzer, H. (1986). *The Fertility Awareness Handbook.* London: Thorsons.

Lev, A. I. (2004). *Transgender Emergence.* Binghamton, NY: Haworth Clinical Practice Press.

Litvinoff, S. (1999). *Sex in Loving Relationships*. London: Vermillion.

Loulan, J. (1987). *Lesbian Passion*. Duluth, MN: Spinsters Ink.

Myss, C. (1997). *Anatomy of the Spirit*. New York: Bantam.

Newman, F. (1999). *The Whole Lesbian Sex Book*. San Francisco, CA: Cleis Press.

Some, S. (1999). *The Spirit of Intimacy: Ancient Teachings in the Ways of Relationships*. New York: HarperCollins.

Villarosa, L. (Ed.) (1994). *Body & Soul: The Black Women's Guide to Physical Health and Emotional Well-Being*. New York: Harper Perennial.

REFERENCES

Amnesty International (2005). UK: New poll finds a third of people believe women who flirt partially responsible for being raped. www.amnesty. org.uk/news_details.asp?NewsID=16618. Accessed 6 December 2011.

Attwood, F. (Ed.) (2010). *Porn.Com: Making Sense of Online Pornography.* New York: Peter Lang.

Bader, E., & Pearson, P. (1998). *In Quest of the Mythical Mate: A Developmental Approach to Diagnosis and Treatment in Couples Therapy.* Florence, KY: Brunner-Mazel.

Bancroft, J. (1989). *Human Sexuality and its Problems.* Philadelphia, PA: Churchill Livingstone.

Banks, S. (2011). Understanding despair, denial, power and emotions in the context of climate change. In *Transformations.* Winter 2011/2012.

Banyard, K. (2010). Sex, lies and videotapes. *The Big Issue,* March 8–14.

Bass, E., & Davis, L. (1990). *The Courage to Heal.* London: Harper & Row.

Basson, R. (2001). Female sexual response: the role of drugs in the management of sexual dysfunction. *Obstetric Gynaecology, 98*: 350–353.

Batmanghelidjh, C. (2007). *Shattered Lives.* London: Jessica Kingsley.

BBC News (2011). Rape crime figure differences revealed. www.bbc.co. uk/news/uk-14844985. Accessed 6 December 2011.

Bennett, J., & Pope, A. (2008). *The Pill.* New South Wales, Australia: Allen & Unwin.

Berne, E. (1961). *Transactional Analysis in Psychotherapy.* MN: Condor Books.

Biddulph, S. (2004). *Manhood.* London: Vermillion.

Bowlby, J. (1988). *A Secure Base.* Abingdon: Routledge.

Bowlby, R. (2004). *Fifty Years of Attachment Theory.* London: Karnac.

Boyle, K. (2007). The impact of pornography. Submission to the Equal Opportunities Committee of the Scottish Parliament.

Boynton, P. (2011). Channel 4 sent complaint from practitioners re problem sex broadcasting. www.drpetra.co.uk/blog/channel-4-sent-complaint-from-practitioners-re-problem-sex-broadcasting/. Accessed 27 November 2011.

Bradshaw, J. (2005). *Healing the Shame That Binds You.* Deerfield Beach, FL: Health Communications.

Brown, B. (2010). The power of vulnerability. TED. www.ted.com/talks/lang/eng/brene_brown_on_vulnerability.html. Accessed 12 April 2012.

Budd, J., Evitt, S., Lynn, H., James, A., & Sutton, L. (2003). Getting lippy. Cosmetics, toiletries and the environment. Women's Environmental Network. www.wen.org.uk/wp-content/uploads/cosmetics_norefs.pdf. Accessed 12 March 2011.

Buhner, S. (2004). *The Secret Teachings of Plants.* Rochester, VT: Bear.

Callaway, E. (2009). Human facial expressions aren't universal. www.newscientist.com/article/dn17605-human-facial-expressions-arent-universal.html. Accessed 19 March 2010.

Cancer Research UK (2008). Prostate cancer – UK incidence statistics. www.info.cancerresearchuk.org/cancerstats/types/prostate/incidence/. Accessed 9 August 2009.

Cardozo, L. (2011). www.guardian.co.uk/lifeandstyle/2011/feb/27/labiaplasty-surgery- labia-vagina-pornography?intcmp=239. Accessed 11 December 2011.

Carnes, P. (2001). *Out of the Shadows.* Center City, MN: Hazelden.

Carnes, P., Delmonico, D., & Griffin, E. (2007). *In The Shadows of the Net.* Center City, MN: Hazelden.

Carrellas, B. (2007). *Urban Tantra.* New York: Celestial Arts.

Carter, H. (2009). 1 in 3 teenage girls tell of sexual abuse by their boyfriends. The *Guardian.* www.guardian.co.uk/society/2009/sep/01/teenage-sexual-abuse-nspcc-report. Accessed 1 September 2009.

Cass, V. (1979). Homosexual identity formation: a theoretical model. *Journal of Homosexuality,* 4(3): 219–235.

Centre for Psychosexual Health. www.psychosexualhealth.org.uk. Accessed 6 April 2012.

Centre for Sex Positive Culture. www.sexpositiveculture.org/. Accessed 11 May 2011.

CER (2006). "Rape of a female" – long-term national recorded crime trend. www.cer.truthaboutrape.co.uk/3.html. Accessed 7 December 2011.

Chalker, R. (2000). *The Clitoral Truth.* New York: Seven Stories.

Chia, M., & Abrams, D. (2002a). *The Multi Orgasmic Man.* London: Thorsons.

Chia, M., & Abrams, D. (2002b). *The Multi Orgasmic Couple.* London: Thorsons.

Chia, M., & Carlton Abrams, R. (2005). *The Multi Orgasmic Woman.* Emmaus, PA: Rodale.

Chugani, H. T., Behen, M. E., Muzik, O., Juhász, C., Nagy, F., & Chugani, D. C. (2001). Local brain functional activity following early deprivation: a study of postinstitutionalized Romanian orphans. *NeuroImage,* *14:* 1290–1301. Accessed at: www.keck.ucsf.edu/~houde/coleman/chugani.pdf. 20 March 2010.

College of Sexual and Relationship Therapists. www.cosrt.org.uk. Accessed 16 March 2012.

Conflict Resolution Network, The (2012). www.crnhq.org. Accessed 22 February 2012.

Cormier-Otaño, O. (2011a). Intimacy, desire, asexualities. Unpublished paper.

Cormier-Otaño, O. (2011b). Doing without: a grounded theory approach to exploring asexuality. Unpublished paper.

Crenshaw, T. (1997). *The Alchemy of Love and Lust.* New York: Pocket Books.

Department of Health. NHS contraceptive services England 1999–2000. www.dh.gov.uk/en/Publicationsandstatistics/Publications/PublicationsStatistics/DH_4009628. Accessed 16 March 2012.

Department of Health (2009). Abortion statistics, England and Wales. www.dh.gov.uk/en/Publicationsandstatistics/Publications/PublicationsStatistics/DH_116039. Accessed 3 October 2011.

Department of Health (2010). *Sexual Violence Against Women subgroup Report.* www.dh.gov.uk/en/Publichealth/Healthimprovement/ViolenceagainstWomenandChildren/DH_104747. Accessed 18 May 2011.

Diamond, L. (2008). *Sexual Fluidity.* Boston, MA: Harvard University Press.

DiGangi, J., & Norin, H. (2002). *Pretty Nasty: Phthalates in European Cosmetic Products.* Healthcare without Harm.

Dines, G. (2010). *Pornland*. Boston, MA: Beacon Press.

Disabilities-r-us. (1997). www.disabilities-r-us.com/sexuality. Accessed 15 March 2012.

Disability Directory of Disabled Information Aids and Mobility Services. www.ableize.com. Accessed 15 March 2012.

Ekman, P. (1980). *The Face of Man: Expressions of Universal Emotions in a New Guinea Village*. New York: Garland STPM Press.

Elworthy, S. (1991). *Power and Sex*. London: Virago.

End Violence Against Women (2007). Female genital mutilation. www. endviolenceagainstwomen.org.uk/pages/female_genital_mutilation. html. Accessed 6 December 2011.

Erikson, E. (1959). *Identity and the Life Cycle*. Madison, CT: International Universities Press.

Family Education Trust (2003). Lessons in Dutch mythology. www. famyouth.org.uk/pdfs/LDM.pdf. Accessed 30 March 2012.

Family Lives (2011). www.besomeonetotell.org.uk/index.php?id=209. Accessed 18 May 2011.

Family Planning Association (FPA) (2007). Contraception: patterns of use factsheet. www.fpa.org.uk/professionals/factsheets/contraception-patternsofuse. Accessed 3 October 2011.

Family Planning Association (FPA) (2012). www.fpa.org.uk. Accessed 15 March 2012.

Farley, M., Bindel, J., & Golding, J. M. (2009). *Men Who Buy Sex, Who They Buy and What They Know*. London: Eaves.

Farmer, E. (2009). www.nspcc.org.uk/Inform/newsandevents/conferencereports/sexual_bullying_why_problem_wdf69255.pdf. Accessed 23 September 2011.

Federation of Feminist Women's Health Centers (FFWHC) (1995). *A New View of a Woman's Body*. Los Angeles, CA: Feminist Health Press.

Feminist Women's Health Center (2011). www.fwhc.org. Accessed 16 March 2012.

Fertility UK (2002). www.fertilityuk.org. Accessed 16 March 2012.

Frank-Herrmann, P., Hell, J., Gnoth, C., Toledo, E., Baur, S., Pyper, C., Jenetzky, E., Strowitzki, T., & Freundl, G. (2007). The effectiveness of a fertility awareness based method to avoid pregnancy in relation to a couple's sexual behaviour during the fertile time: a prospective longitudinal study. *Human Reproduction*, 22(5): 1310–1319. www.humrep. oxfordjournals.org/content/22/5/1310. Accessed 12 December 2011.

Friday, N. (1994). *Forbidden Flowers: More Women's Sexual Fantasies*. New York: Pocket Books.

Gastaldo, E. (2011). Contraceptive shot may double HIV risk. Newser. www.newser.com/story/130125/contraceptive-shot-may-double-hiv-risk.html?utm_source=part&utm_medium=inbox&utm_campaign= newser. Accessed 4 October 2011.

Geraghty, A. (2003). *How Loving Relationships Work.* London: Vega.

Gerhardt, S. (2004). *Why Love Matters.* Hove: Brunner-Routledge.

Gerhardt, S. (2010). *The Selfish Society.* London: Simon & Schuster.

Goldhor Lerner, H. (1990). *The Dance of Intimacy.* Ontario, Canada: Pandora.

Goodman, A. (1998). *Sexual Addiction: An Integrated Approach.* Madison, CT: International Universities Press.

Green, S., & Flemons, D. (2004). *Quickies Handbook of Brief Sex Therapy.* New York: W. W. Norton.

Haines, S. (1999). *The Survivor's Guide to Sex.* San Fransisco, CA: Cleis Press.

Havens, The (2012). www.thehavens.co.uk. Accessed 16 March 2012.

Hawton, K. (1985). *Sex Therapy: A Practical Guide.* Oxford: Oxford Medical Press.

Health Protection Agency (2009). *Contraception and Sexual Health 2008–2009.* www.ons.gov.uk/ons/search/index.html?newquery= contraception+and+sexual+health. Accessed 10 January 2013.

Health Protection Agency (2011). *Regional Trends Online Tables, 06: Health and Care.* www.ons.gov.uk/ons/search/index.html?newquery+HIV+ 2011. Accessed 15 March 2012.

Heinman, J., & LoPiccolo, J. (1998). *Becoming Orgasmic: A Sexual and Personal Growth Programme for Women.* London: Piatkus.

Hendrix, H. (1993). *Getting the Love You Want: A Guide for Couples.* London: Pocket Books.

Hendrix, H. (1995). *Keeping the Love You Find.* London: Pocket Books.

Herman, J. (1993). *Trauma and Recovery.* New York: Basic Books.

Hillier, S. (2008). Hillier Research Group. Magee - Womens Research Institute and Foundation. www.mwrif.org/194/hillier-lab. Accessed 15 March 2012.

Hite, S. (1976). *The Hite Report.* New York: Dell.

Hite, S. (1994). *The Hite Report on the Family.* London: Bloomsbury.

Holden, M. (2008). Rape conviction rate to be improved. Reuters. www.uk.reuters.com/article/domesticNews/idUKL0811903620080709. Accessed 19 January 2009.

Hughes, D. M. (2000). In the shadows: promoting prosperity or undermining stability? *Journal of International Affairs, 53*(2): 625–651.

International Prostitutes Collective (2012). www.prostitutescollective. net/. Accessed 6 January 2012.

Irwin, R. (2002). *Psychosexual Nursing*. London: Whurr.

Kahr, B. (2007). *Sex and the Psyche*. New York: Penguin.

Karpman, S. (1968). Fairy tales and script drama analysis. *Transactional Analysis Bulletin*, 7(26): 39–43. See also: www.karpmandramatriangle. com/. Accessed 11 January 2012.

Kaufman, G., & Raphael, L. (1996). *Coming Out of Shame*. New York: Doubleday.

Kelly, R., & Maxted, F. (2005). *The Survivors Guide*. Rugby: RoSA.

Kessler, D. A. (2010). Obesity: the killer combination of salt, fat and sugar. *Guardian Weekend Magazine*. 13 March.

Kinsey, A., Wardell, P., & Martin, C. (1948). *Sexual Behaviour in the Human Male*. Philadelphia, PA: W. B. Saunders.

Kinsey, A., Wardell, P., & Martin, C. (1953). *Sexual Behaviour in the Human Female*. Philadelphia, PA: W. B. Saunders.

Kitzinger, S. (1985). *Women's Experience of Sex*. New York: Penguin.

Komisaruk, B., Beyer-Flores, C., & Whipple, B. (2006). *The Science of Orgasm*. Baltimore, MD: Johns Hopkins University Press.

Kort, J. (2003). *10 Smart Things Gay Men Can Do To Improve Their Lives*. Los Angeles, CA: Alyson Books.

Kort, J. (2011). www.joekort.com. Accessed 30 March 2012.

Laffy, C. (2001). Developing a humanistic model of psychosexual therapy. *Self and Society*, 29(2): 5–11.

Lee, R. G. (2008). *The Secret Language of Intimacy*. Perth, Western Australia: Gestalt Press.

Levine, P. (1997). *Waking the Tiger*. Berkeley, CA: North Atlantic Books.

Lew, M. (2004). *Victims No Longer*. New York: Harper Collins.

Lightwoman, L. (2004). *Tantra*. London: Piatkus.

Love, P., & Robinson, J. (1995). *Hot Monogamy*. New York: Plume, Penguin.

Macy, J., & Young Brown, M. (1998). *Coming Back to Life*. Canada: New Society.

Maltz, W. (1991). *The Sexual Healing Journey*. New York: HarperCollins.

Maltz, W. (2010). The porn trap. *Therapy Today*, 21(1): www.therapy today.net/article/show/1665/. Acessed 14 January 2013.

Mankind. www.mankindcounselling.org.uk/. Accessed 6 December 2011.

Martin-Sperry, C. (2004). *Couples and Sex*. London: Radcliffe Medical Press.

Masters, W. H., & Johnson, V. E. (1966). *Human Sexual Responses*. New York: Little, Brown.

Masters, W., Johnson, V., & Kolodny, R. (1994). *Heterosexuality*. London: Thorsons.

McGilchrist, I. (2009). *The Master and His Emissary: The Divided Brain and the Making of the Western World*. New Haven, CT: Yale University Press.

McKee, A., Albury, K., & Lumby, C. (2008). *The Porn Report*. Melbourne, Australia: Melbourne University Press.

Miller, A. (1987). *For Your Own Good: Roots of Violence in Childrearing*. London: Virago.

Miller, A. (1991). *Thou Shalt Not Be Aware*. London: Pluto Press.

Miller, A. (2006). *The Body Never Lies: The Lingering Effects of Cruel Parenting*. New York: W. W. Norton.

Miss Naked Beauty (Channel 4 TV show) (2008). www.channel4.com/life/microsites/M/missnakedbeauty/episodes/gallery_4_episode_2.html. Accessed 19 January 2009.

Moore, J. (2008). The jab that can stop cancer. www.channel4.com/news/articles/dispatches/the+jab+that+can+stop+cancer/2346072.html. Accessed 24 January 2012.

Moran, C. (2011). *How to Be a Woman*. London: Ebury Press.

Morin, J. (1996). *The Erotic Mind*. New York: Harper Collins.

My pleasure (2000). www.mypleasure.com. Accessed 15 March 2012.

Nathanson, D. (1992). *Shame and Pride: Affect and the Birth of Self*. New York: W. W. Norton.

National Aids Trust (2011). www.hivaware.org.uk. Accessed 6 January 2012.

National Statistics Online. www.statistics.gov.uk. Accessed 15 March 2012.

Northrup, C. (1995). *Women's Bodies, Women's Wisdom*. London: Piatkus.

Northrup, C. (2003). *The Wisdom of the Menopause*. New York: Bantam.

National Society for the Prevention of Cruelty to Children (NSPCC) (2009). Children talking to ChildLine about sexual abuse. www.nspcc.org.uk/Inform/publications/casenotes/children_talking_to_childline_about_sexual_abuse_wda69414.html. Accessed 6 December 2011.

Odent, M. (1999). *The Scientification of Love*. London: Free Association Books.

O'Dwyer, K. (2011). Can we learn how to love? An exploration of Eric Fromm's *The Art of Loving*. *Self and Society*, *39*(2): 36–47.

Office for National Statistics (2011). www.ons.gov.uk/ons/search/index.html?newquery=Omnibus+survey+reports+on+contraception+and+sexual+health. Accessed 3 October 2011.

Office of Public Sector Information (2003). *Sexual Offences Act*. www. opsi.gov.uk/ACTS/acts2003/en/ukpgaen_20030042_en_1. Accessed 19 January 2009.

Panksepp, J. (1998). *Affective Neuroscience*. New York: Oxford University Press.

Papenfuss, M. (2012). LA porn condom law starts today. www.newser. com/story/141045/la-porn-condom-law-starts-today.html?utm_ source=part&utm_medium=inbox&utm_campaign=newser. Accessed 5 March 2012.

Parentlineplus (2011). www.besomeonetotell.org.uk/index.php?id=209. Accessed 18 May 2011.

Perel, E. (2007). *Mating in Captivity*. London: Hodder.

Pert, C. (1998). *Molecules of Emotion*. New York: Simon and Schuster.

Rape Crisis Statistics (2004–2012). www.rapecrisis.org.uk/Statistics2.php. Accessed 6 December 2011.

Redgrave, K., & Limmer, M. (2005). www.healthyschools.gov.uk/ Uploads/Resources/6e814e06–3939–4fe0-b20a-d3894a4e1010/Alcohol %20and%20Sexual%20Health%20%202004.pdf. Accessed 24 January 2009.

Research Development and Statistics (CRCSG), Home Office. Research and Statistics (2003). www.homeoffice.gov.uk/science-research/ research-statistics/. Accessed 7 December 2011.

Richardson, A. (2009). *The Sex Education Show vs Pornography*. Channel 4 TV. http://sexexperienceuk.channel4.com/sexeducation. Acessed 16 March 2012.

Richardson, A. (2010). *The Sex Education Show*, Season 3, Episode 1. Channel 4 TV. http://sexexperienceuk.channel4.com/sexeducation. Acessed 16 March 2012.

Rose, S. (1999). *The Chemistry of Life*. New York: Penguin.

Roth, G. (1993). *Feeding the Hungry Heart: The Experience of Compulsive Eating*. New York: Plume.

Rothschild, B. (2000). *The Body Remembers*. New York: Norton.

Ruffell, L. (2011). www.lizzieruffell.co.uk . Accessed 16 March 2012.

Schnarch, D. (1998). *Passionate Marriage*. New York: Owl Books.

Schnarch, D. (2002). *Resurrecting Sex*. New York: HarperCollins.

Shapiro, R. (1987). *Contraception: A Practical and Political Guide*. London: Virago.

Sherwin, A. (2011). Sex isn't such a straight choice anymore for Brits. *i Newspaper*, 29 September.

Slater, N. (1993). *Real Fast Food*. New York: Penguin.

Spokz. www.spokz.co.uk. Accessed 16 March 2012.

Sprinkle, A. www.anniesprinkle.org/. Accessed 11 December 2011.

Starhawk (1990). *Truth or Dare*. New York: HarperCollins.

Sunderland, M. (2007). *What Every Parent Needs to Know*. London: Dorling Kindersley.

Survivors UK (2012). www.survivorsuk.org/. Accessed 30 March 2012.

Swami, V., & Furnham, A. (2008). *The Psychology of Physical Attraction*. London: Routledge.

Terrence Higgins Trust. www.tht.org.uk/informationresources/facts andstatistics/uk/. Accessed 3 October 2011.

Tomljenovic, L. (2011). Gardasil vaccination: evaluating the risks versus benefits. Sane Vax. www.sanevax.org/wp-content/uploads/2011/02/Gardasil-vaccination-risks-vs-benefits-FINAL1221.pdf. Accessed 11 March 2012.

Truth About Rape Campaign. (2012). www.truthaboutrape.co.uk/4598.html. Accessed 30 March 2012.

UC Davis student health and counseling services (2011). www.health center.ucdavis.edu/topics/contraception/efficacy.html. Accessed 12 December 2011.

UK Association of Humanistic Psychology Practitioners. www.ahpp.org. Accessed 12 April 2012.

Walter, N. (2010). *Living Dolls*. London: Virago.

Weiss, R. (2005). *Cruise Control: Understanding Sex Addiction in Gay Men*. New York: Alyson Books.

Whipple, B., & Brash-McGreer, K. (1997). Management of female sexual dysfunction. In: M. L. Sipski & C. J. Alexander (Eds.), *Sexual Function in People with Disability and Chronic Illness* (pp. 509–534). New York: Aspen.

Women's Environmental Network (2006). www.wen.org.uk/cosmetics/facts.htm. Accessed 26 January 2009.

Women's Health (2012). Infertility. www.womens-health.co.uk/infertility 4.asp. Accessed 16 March 2012.

World Health Organisation (2009). Eight-year trend shows new HIV infections down by 17%—most progress seen in sub-Saharan Africa. www.unaids.org/en/media/unaids/contentassets/dataimport/pub/pressrelease/2009/20091124_pr_epiupdate_en.pdf. Accessed 3 October 2011.

Zilbergeld, B. (1992). *The New Male Sexuality*. New York: Bantam.

INDEX